# PREMED MONDAYS

*52 Letters of Mentorship
to a Future Doctor*

BY DALE OKORODUDU, MD

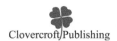

Clovercroft Publishing

PreMed Mondays

Published by Clovercroft Publishing, Franklin, Tennessee

Edited by Tammy Kling and Christy Callahan

Cover Design by Debbie Manning Sheppard

Interior Design by Suzanne Lawing

ISBN: 978-1-945507-98-4

Printed in the United States of America

**To my wife & children**
*I love you. The only reason I can do the things I do is because of your support. On behalf of every individual who will read this book, thank you for making it possible for me to share my gifts with the world.*

**To my greatest physician mentors:**
**Dr. Ellis Ingram & Dr. Cedric Bright**
*The two of you have mentored me as a physician and as a human. Your dedication to serving others has influenced me more than you can imagine. I am grateful to have mentors such you.*

**To my premedical friends**
*Everyone deserves a mentor. I'd love to walk this journey with you.*

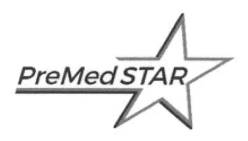

Before we begin our journey together, please join PreMedSTAR.com, the free online community for premedical students! The best support you will receive on the road to medical school will be from your fellow premeds. Take a moment to download the free app in your app store.

**www.PreMedSTAR.com**

# CONTENTS

*My mentor said to me, "Let's go do it!" Not you go do it.*
*How powerful it is when someone says, "Let's."*

—JIM ROHN

# Week 1

# INTRODUCTION

*To my premedical friend:*

I have been asked why I would take the time to write a book of fifty-two letters to premedical students, the majority of whom I will never meet. Where do I begin? I suppose I should share my heart with you, and my passion for mentoring.

Outside of family, my first great mentor was Dr. Ellis Ingram. During my premedical years, he frequently invited my friends and me to chat at a coffee shop. Back then I didn't know any better, and always turned down his invitation. I failed to appreciate how valuable the guidance of somebody of his stature would be in my life. Dr. Ingram was very well respected not only on our campus, but across the nation. As an accomplished medical doctor and mentor, he had been awarded the Presidential Award for Mentoring in Sciences. Perhaps I thought a professor like him wouldn't truly care about a student like me. But I was wrong.

One day, for reasons unknown, I came to my senses and took Dr. Ingram up on his invitation. We met at his office, and he took me on a tour of the entire medical school. For the first time, I had a palpable experience that truly allowed me to envision what medical school might be like. Dr. Ingram even walked me through the admissions office and personally introduced me to every individual. At the end of the VIP tour, he took me directly into the dean of the medical school's office for an unscheduled, yet welcomed, introduction. I will never forget that day and how much it meant to me.

Since then, I have desired to impact the lives of others in a similar fashion. I ended up going to that medical school, largely because of Dr. Ingram, and was privileged to gain further mentoring experience under his tutelage. In a sense, he handed me a torch that he expected to burn even brighter in my hands. Via DiverseMedicine Inc., Black Men in White Coats, and PreMed STAR, I have been blessed to work with wonderful doctors who share my passion, and together we have watched many of our mentees go on to do outstanding things. These mentees are the reason I wrote the fifty-two letters in this book. Now, I would like to share them with you.

Though I may not be there in person, I would love to walk your journey with you. I remember the path to medical school. The terrain was rocky at times, and when I needed someone to provide guidance, I was blessed to find that person. I hope to be such a person for you, and that is the reason why I wrote PreMed Mondays.

Within the pages of this book you will always have somebody to turn to. These fifty-two letters are designed to guide you along your premedical path to success. You will benefit most by doing two things: First, ask one of your premedical friends to be your accountability buddy and review each letter with him or her. Second, commit yourself to reading one letter every Monday morning. To be sure you don't forget, take thirty seconds right now to set a recurrent Monday morning alarm called "PreMed Monday."

Throughout this book, you will find letters from me pertaining to concepts that are often not taught to premedical students. Concepts such as success, vision, discipline, belief, and your "why" are all essential for you to perform well, not only as a doctor, but as a person. My desire is to add value to your life as a human, not just as a physician. Please do not overlook these concepts, because they are absolutely necessary for you to be your best.

Every week, I will challenge you to do something. These assignments will take minimal effort, but the future rewards will be tremendous. This week I challenge you to find your premedical accountability buddy. There are few things as valuable as a good friend. If you can find one who will also hold you accountable along your journey, amazing things are in store for you!

Thank you for allowing me to join you on your journey. At the end of the year, I would love it if you would contact me and let me know how you are doing.

I'm praying for your success, and look forward to our time together next Monday.

*Dr. Dale*

## THIS WEEK'S ASSIGNMENT
• Find a premedical accountability buddy.

# Week 2

# FIVE THINGS I WISH I HAD KNOWN BEFORE BECOMING A MEDICAL DOCTOR

*To my premedical friend:*

Life as a medical doctor is not exactly what I thought it would be. As a premedical student, I thought I had done sufficient research about the field of medicine to have a great grasp of what my future would look like. I watched videos, read articles, and spoke with physicians. At the end of the day, I still didn't appreciate certain things pertaining to life as a medical doctor until I became one. Now, in retrospect, I can share with you the things I wish I had known when I was in your position. Here are five of the most important.

1) **This is the best job in the world.** I believe this is true because as a doctor, you get to connect with people on a unique level. There are few career fields in which people completely open up about their lives to a stranger. They

will tell you their deepest secrets, literally trusting you with their lives. I can't even begin to tell you how many times a patient's life was in jeopardy and I was told, "Dr. Dale, just do whatever you think is right." That is trusting beyond all borders. There is nothing quite like it, and with every patient encounter, I am reminded that it is an honor and privilege to wear the white coat.

2) **The journey to become a medical doctor isn't hard— it's very hard.** As it is with other privileges, you must earn the right to wear the white coat. If you are going to care for the lives of others, you must be fully prepared. I want you to understand that going through medical school, residency, fellowship, then practice is not just hard, it is very hard. Along this journey, you will have ups and downs, but in the end, your ups will win. The journey to get here is harder than you can imagine; however, it's completely worth it.

3) **Every day is rewarding.** When you become a medical doctor, you will have friends who do not like their jobs. They'll complain about how mundane it is and why they deserve more money, and then tell you they're looking for other jobs. Many of them will wake up and go to a job that they hate. Since I earned my MD, to this day, that has never been the case for me. Yes, there are aspects of medicine I personally could do without, but regarding the field and my job as a whole, I love every single day!

4) **We are all human.** When you become a doctor, you'll come to understand the respect and reverence others have for our field. This is great, but the downside is they sometimes forget physicians are fallible human beings too. More than likely, there will be a day in your career when you will make a major mistake which leads to a

serious negative patient outcome. As physicians, we must stay humble and remember that we are simply human. Our job is to always do our best. As long as we're doing that, our patients will appreciate us.

5) **You can do it.** Now, I don't want to be misleading and suggest to you that everyone can become a medical doctor, because that's not the case. There is a baseline level of intellect you must have, and for the most part, if you are in college, you've likely crossed that threshold. Beyond that, whether or not you succeed in becoming a medical doctor is determined by your G.R.I.N.D. Nine times out of ten, the person who worked hard to prepare will outperform the person who depended on raw talent. By reading *PreMed Mondays* you are preparing, and I suspect that your grind extends beyond this book. That is why I believe that you (not everyone else—I am writing to you) can do it!

My challenge to you this week is to spend some time with your accountability buddy discussing what things make a job rewarding for you, and whether or not the medical field can provide them.

I'd love to hear how your challenge went. Tweet me @DoctorDaleMD #PreMedMondays. I continue to pray for your success, and I look forward to our time together next Monday.

*Dr. Dale*

### THIS WEEK'S ASSIGNMENT
- What makes a job rewarding for you?
- Can the medical field provide those things for you?
- Discuss your answers with your accountability buddy.

# Week 3

# FIVE WAYS TO KNOW MEDICINE IS THE RIGHT CAREER FOR YOU

*To my premedical friend:*

In the age of information and technology, there are numerous careers for students to choose from. They seem to be infinite, but you are reading this letter because you believe medicine is the right one for you. How do you know that? I'd like to share five simple ways that can help you determine if medicine is the right career for you.

1) **You want to help people.** This statement is often said to be cliché, but cliché does not preclude the truth. Everybody in the field of medicine should desire to help people. If this desire isn't in you, then medicine isn't the right field for you. As a physician, when you see another human-being sick and suffering, your initial instinct is to help them, even if you don't have the resources to do so. This is the first key to knowing that medicine is

the right career for you. Ask yourself, *When I see people hurting, do I want to make them feel better?*

2) **You are curious.** The field of medicine is ever-changing, and medical doctors are lifelong learners. At our core, there is an unquenchable curiosity to learn why the human body works the way that it does and how to heal its ailments. This curiosity drives our search for knowledge, which we desire to use for good. Without curiosity, your career as a physician can become a burden.

3) **You are patient.** The journey to become a medical doctor is a long one. To earn the privilege of caring for human life, you must invest the necessary time to master the art and science of medicine. Nobody wants to be taken care of by a physician who only trained for one year. Your patients put their care in your hands. This is a big responsibility, and in order to take it on, you must exercise patience on multiple levels.

4) **You've been exposed to it and you still want to do it.** I can't emphasize this enough. You must shadow doctors and spend time in real medical environments. Don't think modern television paints an accurate picture of the physician lifestyle. You need to ask real physicians what their life is like in order to get a true understanding of the field you are pursuing. If you've spent adequate time in medical environments, have discussed the lifestyle with physicians, and are still interested in becoming a doctor, then this just might be the field for you.

5) **Nothing else excites you this way.** At the end of the day, there's a certain feeling we get from what we do as physicians. It's a feeling of purpose and belonging. Medicine is a true calling, and when your name is on its list, you

can feel it. You'll know because nothing else makes you feel the same way. It's kind of like love. When you meet that perfect individual, you just know it.

My challenge to you this week is to go through these five items, and evaluate if medicine is right for you. Discuss your thoughts with your accountability buddy.

I'd love to hear how your challenge went. Tweet me @DoctorDaleMD #PreMedMondays. I continue to pray for your success, and I look forward to our time together next Monday.

*Dr. Dale*

## THIS WEEK'S ASSIGNMENT

- Go through these five items, and ask yourself, "Is medicine right for me?"
- Discuss your thoughts with your accountability buddy.

# Week 4

# FIVE WAYS TO STAY MOTIVATED AS A PREMED

*To my premedical friend:*

During this journey, there will be days when you want to quit. You might make a bad grade, miss too many parties, or have personal issues. Just because you are a premed student does not mean life will stop and wait for you. Being a premedical student is challenging, and only the strong survive. So, stay strong!

Here are five ways for you to stay motivated during difficult times as a premed student:

1) **Make flyers (or use Post-it notes) of encouraging and inspiring quotes and post them on your wall.** You want your home, workspace, and study environment to be filled with positivity. Everywhere you look, you should be inspired. Phrases such as, "Failure is not an option!" and, "Go get that medical degree!" are examples of notes you can stick on a board in your room to help keep you

motivated.

2) **Have dinner at least once a week with a premed friend.** Encourage one another to work hard and continue along the path. It is much easier to be successful when you are on the journey with somebody else. Commit to having dinner together on the same day each week.

3) **Watch medical shows on TV.** Allow yourself to fantasize about what life will be like when you are wearing your white coat. Put yourself in the main character's role and be the doctor. Life in medicine isn't quite as glamorous as the sitcoms, but allow your imagination to take you there.

4) **Join PreMed STAR.com.** There's nothing like being in a community with thousands of people who share the same goal. These students are facing the same ups and downs that you are. Connecting with other premeds is exciting and can keep you motivated.

5) **Set goals.** Keep your eyes on the medical school admission prize, but also set smaller, more frequent goals. Each time you accomplish one, give yourself a pat on the back and a treat of some sort. Look back at your successes to realize that you have what it takes to keep going. At times it can seem overwhelming, but just choose one goal to start with. Take a baby step.

My challenge to you this week is to post something inspirational on your wall.

I'd love to see what you posted. Take a photo of it and tweet me @DoctorDaleMD #PreMedMondays. I continue to pray for your success, and I look forward to our time together next Monday.

*Dr. Dale*

## THIS WEEK'S ASSIGNMENT
• Post something inspirational on your wall to help keep you motivated.

*My mother said to me, 'If you are a soldier, you will become a general. If you are a monk, you will become the Pope." Instead, I was a painter, and became Picasso.*

—PABLO PICASSO

# Week 5

# SUCCESS AND PERSONAL DEVELOPMENT

*To my premedical friend:*

Isn't success an interesting concept? Everybody wants it, yet we can't agree on a definition for it. What is your definition of success? How do you measure it? Certainly, there are many aspects to this nebulous concept, but I am convinced that the best way to measure success is by how you have helped others.

I want to caution you about the "hedonic treadmill." This phrase is used to describe a reality that unfortunately too many physicians are stuck in. This "reality" is when we want something so bad that we work endlessly to get it. When we do get it, we become unimpressed and want the next hot thing. Money, cars, big houses—those things are all benign in and of themselves, but if you use them as a gauge for success, you'll find yourself fighting off a bitter and insidious cancer that will drive you into a state of perpetual discontentment.

Before you begin medical school, it is important that you

set your own priorities. If you don't, society will set them for you. And truth be told, society doesn't care about your feelings. Trust me when I say this: You do not want to get on the hedonic treadmill. It will run you to death. To avoid it, you must define your own values and adhere to them.

Pouring your heart out to serve and help others will satisfy you beyond any material possession. This joy is amazing, and it never gets old. That's what being a doctor is all about—serving others. It's the heart of our medical profession. The white coat isn't about power and respect; it's about servitude. As you walk this premedical journey, always remember that your ultimate success will be based on what you give, and not what you receive.

My challenge to you this week is to evaluate how you define true success. Jot down some notes pertaining to this and discuss it with your accountability buddy.

I'd love to hear how your challenge went. Tweet me @DoctorDaleMD #PreMedMondays. I continue to pray for your success, and I look forward to our time together next Monday.

*Dr. Dale*

## THIS WEEK'S ASSIGNMENT
• How do you define true success?
• Discuss your definition with your accountability buddy.

# Week 6

# FIVE THINGS THAT CAN PREVENT YOU FROM BECOMING A MEDICAL DOCTOR

*To my premedical friend:*

Just because you want something does not mean you'll get it. In the United States, there are a lot more students applying to medical school than getting in. Often, mentors (myself included) and advisors focus on the things premeds should do in order to get into medical school. However, it's just as important to recognize the things that will prevent you from becoming a doctor.

1) **Lack of confidence.** This is the most common reason why premedical students never achieve their goal of getting into medical school. Often, students begin college with a burning passion for medicine, which leads to a feeling of invincibility. In their minds, the premed journey will be a breeze and they'll be docs in no time. That's true until the unthinkable happens. They fail an exam.

This one thing has irreversibly damaged the confidence of too many premeds. Do not let this happen to you! We all perform poorly at one time or another. You must bounce back and maintain your confidence with humility. Lack of confidence is the number one reason most premedical students never become medical students.

2) **Overconfidence.** Perhaps a better way to say this would be having too much pride. I know I just told you that the number one problem was lack of confidence, and now I'm telling you not to have too much of it. These two things are not mutually exclusive, and you need to know how to balance them. The problem with having too much confidence is that you will never know when to ask for help, and even if you do know when to ask, you might be too prideful to do so. Would you rather be a doctor, or be prideful and not ask anyone for help when needed? I know my answer. What's yours? Don't be one of those premedical students who refuses to ask for help and watches his or her dreams slowly go by the wayside.

3) **Lack of discipline.** Many people have asked me, "What is the key to success as a premedical student?" Well, here is my big secret: You must be extremely disciplined! The premedical journey will demand consistency and time. If you are not disciplined enough to meet these demands, you will not be successful. Disciplined in your study, disciplined in your exercise, disciplined in your faith, disciplined in your diet—all these things matter.

4) **Lack of mentorship.** The truth is, nobody becomes a doctor without a little help from others. Often, the individuals who are weeded out of the premedical journey are those who simply don't know what they need to do to be successful. Yes, the mentorship I am providing to

you in these letters will give you a leg up, but you need more. You must have personal mentors to help get you to your goal!

5) **Lack of resources.** Yes, I'm talking about the things that money can buy. Unfortunately, the reality of the situation is that succeeding as a premedical student requires financial resources—for college tuition, living expenses, and of course, textbooks. Beyond that, there's the MCAT (Medical College Admission Test), medical school applications, and travel costs to your interviews. These things aren't free. There is good news, however. Just because these things cost money doesn't mean it has to be *your* money. There are plenty of resources available to discount or waive the costs for many premedical expenses.

My challenge to you this week is to think of at least one thing with which you could use some help with. Once you've thought of it, ask someone for help. This is a humbling experience, but it's necessary for success in all fields.

I'd love to hear how your challenge went. Tweet me @DoctorDaleMD #PreMedMondays. I continue to pray for your success, and I look forward to our time together next Monday.

*Dr. Dale*

**THIS WEEK'S ASSIGNMENT**
- What could you use help with?
- Ask someone to help you.

2|c

# Week 7

# FIVE REASONS TO CHOOSE YOUR FRIENDS WISELY

*To my premedical friend:*

Who are your best friends? The saying goes, "Show me your five closest friends and I'll tell you who you are." During college, you have the opportunity to build an entirely new group of friends. These individuals will greatly affect the trajectory of your life and success. It's important that you carefully craft your network. Here are five reasons to choose your friends wisely:

1) **They will influence how you spend your time.** For the premedical student, time is worth more than gold. You need as much of it as possible to get ready for medical school. Your non-premedical friends, and even some of your premed friends, may not appreciate how important getting that "A" is. That being the case, you might be pressured to spend your time in ways that won't contribute to your academic success. Your friends need to be

31

respectful of the time you allot toward your goals.

2) **Friends build character.** The nature of a premedical student is to help improve the lives of others. This is a wonderful character trait that you should encourage your friends to foster and develop in themselves. Keep in mind that you can influence the character traits of your friends, and they can do the same for you. Surround yourself with people who challenge you to be better.

3) **Friends are your support system.** Along the premedical journey, you will have some bad days, and you'll need somebody to talk to. It is important that you have close friends in whom you can confide, and who are willing to give you that extra boost of confidence when you are unable to give it to yourself.

4) **People will make judgments about you based on the company you keep.** You don't want to be "guilty by association." If your friends are a group of knuckleheads, people will think you are a knucklehead as well. If your friends are responsible and goal-oriented individuals, people will assume the same of you. I know, this doesn't sound fair, but that's how life works.

5) **Friends are a key source of resources.** Access to resources is extremely important for premedical students. There are always study guides, test prep discounts, or free giveaways circulating in the premed world, but if you don't know about them, you can't take advantage of them. The easiest way to learn about something is by having someone else tell you about it. Your friends need to be "in the know." Just as much as they provide you with resources, you should also contribute to their success by providing resources for them.

My challenge to you this week is to make a list of your five closest friends and write down how they influence you.

I'd love to hear how your challenge went. Tweet me @DoctorDaleMD #PreMedMondays. I continue to pray for your success, and I look forward to our time together next Monday.

*Dr. Dale*

**THIS WEEK'S ASSIGNMENT**
• Who are your five closest friends?
• How do they influence you? Write it down.

# Week 8

# FIVE WAYS TO STAY MENTALLY AND PHYSICALLY HEALTHY AS A PREMED

*To my premedical friend:*

By now, you are surely learning that being a premedical student is not a walk in the park. Life can be very stressful, and it is important that you do your best to keep your mind and body healthy. These five tips will help you do just that!

1) **Have a study plan.** One of your goals as a premedical student is to get good grades. That being the case, it is likely that a decent percentage of your stressors are related to studying. To ease the stress, make sure you have a study plan you can adhere to. Without a solid plan, you'll be making things up as you go. That's not a good idea if you want to minimize stress.

2) **Eat a healthy diet.** The "Freshman 15" isn't a myth! It's

real. During your college years, you will spend an excessive amount of time in campus cafeterias and fast food restaurants. Both places tend to load your belly with sugar and fat. High carbohydrate foods increase fatigue, cause weight gain, and can lead to overall poor performance. Be sure to eat your fair share of fruits and vegetables daily for that organic boost in energy. It's certainly a challenge to do this in college, but if you want to perform with the best of them, you have to eat like the best of them.

3) **Exercise at least three times a week.** Exercising is a great way to increase your energy level. The beat of your heart, sweat on your head, and deep inhalations are all exhilarating. Consider exercising prior to studying in order to enhance your focus. Another great thing about exercising is that it's a great way to socialize with others.

4) **Read a book that has nothing to do with your coursework.** Take some time to fill your brain with something that is irrelevant to your coursework. Reading is good because not only can it be very enjoyable, but it also allows you to work on your reading comprehension, which will be important for your MCAT (Medical College Admissions Test).

5) **It's okay to party.** That's right, I said party. You are in college, so make sure you get some partying in while you are there. Just be sure to stay sober, stay modest, and stay out of trouble.

My challenge to you this week is to head to the gym and get in a good workout with your accountability buddy.

I'd love to see a photo of your workout study break. Tweet me @DoctorDaleMD #PreMedMondays. I continue to pray for your success, and I look forward to our time together next Monday.

*Dr. Dale*

## THIS WEEK'S ASSIGNMENT
• Schedule a time to work out with your accountability buddy.

# Week 9

# VISION AND PERSONAL DEVELOPMENT

*To my premedical friend:*

This week I want to discuss the starting point for success, which is vision.

Every successful person begins his or her journey with a great vision. This must be the case because without it, you have nothing to strive for. Keep in mind however that having a vision is slightly different from having vision. I want you to focus on the latter, having vision.

Two things are needed for someone to have vision.

The first necessity is having an object for your vision. This object is the thing or the goal you are trying to obtain or achieve. It is what you see far off in the distance. It is important that you see this object not as it is, but as it should be.

Here's an example. You dream of becoming a medical doctor. I'm willing to bet that the doctor you desire to become is a phenomenal one—one loved by patients, loved by staff, and loved by students. You see yourself as an exemplary physician. You certainly don't see yourself as a doctor who makes errors and is hated by patients. People who have vision can see things the way they should be.

The second aspect of having vision is the ability to see the path necessary to reach your goal. It will do you no good to envision yourself in a white coat if you do not know how to get there.

Proverbs 29:18 says, "Where there is no vision, the people perish." What an amazing truth! If you do not have vision pertaining to your premedical journey, you will not become a medical doctor. It is also important to realize that you have to believe in this vision and that it has to be your own. If you do it because someone else wants you to do so, then you will be doing yourself and your patients a disservice.

My challenge to you this week is for you to write your vision on a sheet of paper. You can write it in a journal or on a poster to hang on your wall (like I did). Look at it at least once a week (daily if possible). This will motivate you beyond measure.

I'd love to hear how your challenge went. Tweet me @DoctorDaleMD #PreMedMondays. I continue to pray for your success, and I look forward to our time together next Monday.

*Dr. Dale*

## THIS WEEK'S ASSIGNMENT
• Write down your vision—in a journal or on a poster board.
• Look at your vision every day (or at least once a week).

# Week 10

# FIVE MENTORS YOU SHOULD HAVE

*To my premedical friend:*

No one becomes a medical doctor without the help of others. The most expeditious way to accomplish something difficult in life is to have someone show you how they did it. Such individuals can be called mentors. Every premedical student should have mentors. If you don't have at least one, you might as well say goodbye to your dream career. Keep in mind however, you often need more than one mentor to be successful. Having a team of mentors will maximize your chances of achieving your goals. Here are five types of mentors that you should have:

1) **A peer mentor.** Your peer mentor should also be on the premedical journey, but slightly ahead of you. In some situations, the two of you may be in the same grade level, but there should be something that he or she can assist with pertaining to your development. An example of a good peer mentor for a freshman or sophomore would

be an upper-level classman who just gained admission to medical school or one who is preparing to take the MCAT. These individuals are further along the journey than you, but still close enough to empathize with your current reality.

2) **A medical student or physician mentor.** Ideally, if you could have one of each, that would be great. However, I understand that this can be difficult to achieve. It is critical for premedical students to get guidance from somebody who is currently in the position that they wish to attain. This is the individual who will be able to give you the real scoop on medicine. Your medical student or physician mentor will play a key role in providing the realities of the field to you, because believe me when I say that it is nothing like what you see on television. Get the facts!

3) **A research mentor.** Not every premedical student will conduct research, but I highly encourage you to at least try it. Research is a great example of something that you won't know you like until you give it a shot. If you do decide to go for it, be sure to seek out a good mentor, because your experience with this individual will play a role in your feelings toward scientific research.

4) **An academic mentor.** For many, this individual will be your premedical advisor. While this is okay, please keep in mind that an advisor is different from a mentor. It is possible, however, for your advisor to also serve as a mentor. Advisors provide advice, but mentors take a vested interest in your success and walk the journey with you. Try to form a deeper connection with your advisor so that he or she may become more of a mentor. If that is not possible, find another individual, such as a

professor, who knows the nitty-gritty about premedical requirements and how to build a strong application.

5) **A spiritual mentor.** Needless to say, the premedical journey is difficult. You will have many ups and downs. Through all of them, you will need somebody to turn to for the well-being of your spirit. This is the individual who will remind you that there are more important things in life than becoming a medical doctor, but at the same time, he or she will do everything possible to make sure you do become one.

My challenge to you this week is to list these mentor types, then identify who that person is in your life. If you do not have one, consider reaching out to find one.

I'd love to hear how your challenge went. Tweet me @DoctorDaleMD #PreMedMondays. I continue to pray for your success, and I look forward to our time together next Monday.

*Dr. Dale*

## THIS WEEK'S ASSIGNMENT

• Who are your mentors?
• Make a list of people who would be good mentors for you.

*Whoever walks with the wise becomes wise,*
*but companions of fools will suffer harm.*

—PROVERBS 13:20 ESV

# Week 11

# FIVE THINGS TO CONSIDER WHEN CHOOSING A MAJOR

*To my premedical friend:*

Another question I am often asked is what major premedical students should choose. As competitive type "A" personalities, most premeds want to ensure they are on the right path for success. While there are many important reasons to choose the "right" major, I would say the most significant of them is that you want to maintain your sanity. The premedical journey is difficult, and the last thing you want to do is choose a major for the wrong reason. Here are five things to consider when choosing your major:

1) **Major in something you enjoy.** There is a common myth that permeates the premedical world, it's that premedical students must major in biology, chemistry, or biochemistry. This is false. Medical schools don't even require you to major in a science field. As a matter of

fact, many medical schools will look favorably upon you if you major in a non-science field because this demonstrates that you might be a more well-rounded student. Major in something you like and are curious about. You may never get another chance to study it down the line.

2) **You can have more than one major.** It is possible to double major in college, and this can also make you a more attractive candidate for medical school. Double-majoring will allow you to explore more areas that might be of interest to you while in college. It should be noted, however, that if you choose to have a double major, it is likely you will have a tad bit more work to do. But in the end, if two things really interest you, consider majoring in both of them. Just keep in mind that grades matter, so don't overburden yourself.

3) **Don't pick a major just because it's easy.** Certain college majors are thought to be easier than others. If you truly like one of these majors, it is okay to pick that one. But if you are choosing this major only because you think you will get better grades, pick something else. Medical school admissions committees pay attention to majors, and they understand that a 4.0 in a difficult one is not equivalent to a 4.0 in a less challenging major.

4) **Choose something.** It is important to not fall into the trap of remaining undecided for too long. Nobody wants a doctor that is indecisive. It is okay to choose a major and change it down the line, but please, please, please choose something!

5) **Master your major.** If you are going to spend all this time and money in college, then you want to be certain that once you leave, you have mastered your major. Really

take these four, five, or six years to get a good under-standing of it. When you leave college, you want to be somewhat of an expert in this area. Don't just major in it, master it!

My challenge to you this week is to commit to mastering your major! That's all. Just commit to it!

I'd love to hear how your challenge went. Tweet me @DoctorDaleMD #PreMedMondays. I continue to pray for your success, and I look forward to our time together next Monday.

*Dr. Dale*

## THIS WEEK'S ASSIGNMENT
• What major(s) have you chosen?
• What practical steps can you take to master your major(s)?

# Week 12

# FIVE KEYS TO CHOOSING YOUR CLASSES

*To my premedical friend:*

Some premedical students are completely lost when it comes to choosing classes. This is of utmost importance because you must have the proper prerequisites to apply for medical school. Knowing what those classes are early in your undergraduate years is essential. Also, aside from taking the right prerequisites, there are some classes to know about that will help expand your base of knowledge prior to starting medical school. Here are five suggestions to help you choose the best classes and maximize your chances of success:

1) **Meet with your premed advisor.** It is very important to meet with your premedical advisor as soon as you can every semester. Many students fall into the trap of registering for classes because a friend told them to do so. Yes, it is important to seek guidance from your friends,

but please do remember that there are advisors who specialize in keeping you on the right path to success. Your advisors should know what classes you need to take.

2) **Consider a few schools that you might be interested in going to.** As early as your freshman year, you should begin considering which schools might be right for you. An easy way to start is by identifying your state's public medical schools. Go to their websites and see which courses they require for admission. This is important because not all medical schools will require the same courses. The last thing you want is to apply to a medical school just to find out that you were one course short of meeting their requirements.

3) **Balance your course load appropriately.** Sometimes, premedical students try to take too many difficult courses in one semester. While this is commendable, it often leads to a lower grade point average and hinders your ability to master the subject matter. Balancing your course load means having a good mix of difficult and less difficult courses in the same semester, as well as knowing which semesters to take more credit hours.

4) **Talk with upperclassmen.** Let's be real—not all professors are good. Speak with the upperclassmen to learn which professors do the best job teaching their subject matter. It is important to learn the basic sciences well as an undergrad so you'll be prepared for the MCAT and your medical school coursework. Make sure you get into the classes with the best professors.

5) **Have some fun.** Every semester, try to take at least one course that you enjoy. This course may count toward your science GPA or might just be something that you've

wanted to do all your life. For example, how about taking a course on self-defense.

My challenge to you this week is to review the prerequisites for at least one state medical school that you are interested in. Write them down so you'll have them for reference later on.

I'd love to hear how your challenge went. Tweet me @DoctorDaleMD #PreMedMondays. I continue to pray for your success, and I look forward to our time together next Monday.

*Dr. Dale*

### THIS WEEK'S ASSIGNMENT
• What are the prerequisites of a state medical school that you are interested in?
• Write down those prereqs for future reference.

# Week 13

# KNOW YOUR WHY

*To my premedical friend:*

May I ask you a question? Well, it seems I just did. Allow me to ask you another: What is your "why"? Previously, I challenged you to write down your vision on a sheet of paper. Today, I am asking you, What is your "why" for that vision?

I believe that you must understand vision before you can evaluate your "why," but in order for that vision to be brought to fruition, you have to understand why you want it. Your why is your true motivation, the fuel to your fire. This is what gets you up every morning to go to class, even when you've only slept two hours (not because you were out partying but studying of course). This is what will make you study harder than you thought you could for the MCAT and other important tests.

I want you to truly understand your "why" because without a doubt, it is the key element to your success. You will never be successful if you don't know what you want and why you want it. A personal knowledge of these two things is what will allow you to fully invest your time and energy into bringing your vision to fruition.

My why for PreMed Mondays is this: I want the most dedicated and caring premedical students to become our nation's doctors because I believe that we all prosper when society is healthy. In order to read a chapter every week and discuss it with your accountability buddy, you have to be dedicated. Therefore, I believe this book will help the right people, and others will be weeded out. This book will help to ensure that our nation gets the best (not just the smartest) doctors.

My challenge to you this week is to share your "why" with your accountability buddy.

I'd love to hear what your "why" is. Tweet me @DoctorDaleMD #PreMedMondays. I continue to pray for your success, and I look forward to our time together next Monday.

*Dr. Dale*

## THIS WEEK'S ASSIGNMENT
• What is your "why"?
• Share your "why" with your accountability buddy.

# Week 14

# FIVE KEYS TO MAKING STRAIGHT "A"S

*To my premedical friend:*

Whether we like it or not, numbers matter. As a premedical student, your grade point average is probably the most important number of them all. Nowadays, medical schools review applicants in a more holistic fashion. This means they try to view non-numeric traits and experiences of students with as much importance as their GPA and scores.

But let's be real—at the end of the day, numbers still matter. So, during your undergrad years, do the best you can to get straight "A"s. If you've already made some bad grades, it's okay; today is a new day! I know it's easier said than done, but here are five tips to help you accomplish this goal:

1) **Believe you can do it.** First and foremost, you must believe that you are smart enough, as well as resourceful enough, to make straight "A"s. Nobody is going to

give you a 4.0 GPA. You will have to earn it. But before you can earn it, you must believe that you are capable of earning it. Begin every semester by telling yourself that your goal is a 4.0, and that you are capable of achieving it.

2) **Motivate yourself.** One of the best ways to motivate yourself to accomplish anything is to write down your goal in big letters (and/or numbers) and place it in a place that you will see every day. This way you cannot escape your goal. Every morning, it will be there reminding you, 4.0!

3) **Ask others to hold you accountable.** It's very easy to set a goal and not tell anybody about it. If you don't reach that goal, it doesn't matter as much because nobody knew that you failed to reach it. However, if you have others to hold you accountable, then the heat is on. This will push you to work harder, and move you one step closer to getting straight "A"s.

4) **Master study techniques.** It is important that you learn how to study by yourself, as well as with a group. You spend more time with yourself than anybody else, so you need to know how to teach yourself. Group study is also important because that is your opportunity to not only learn from others, but to teach others. By teaching others, you are demonstrating to yourself that you have mastered the material. Ultimately, the key element of studying is to be disciplined. You must make a study schedule and stick to it.

5) **Use your resources.** Perhaps the top resources that all premedical students should use are their professors. Professors have office hours for a reason. They expect

students to come and learn. Make it a habit that one week before every test, you go to your professor's office (during office hours) and ask any questions you may have. Also, utilize your campus tutors. Many schools have free tutors; so anytime there is a particular concept you do not understand, find somebody who can teach you. You can even connect with a study buddy on PreMed STAR. Nowadays, you don't need to be in the same room to learn from one another. You should never go into a test not prepared to score 100 percent.

My challenge to you this week is to make a sign with your semester GPA goal and hang it up in your room.

I'd love to see a photo of your sign with your GPA goal. Tweet me @DoctorDaleMD #PreMedMondays. I continue to pray for your success, and I look forward to our time together next Monday.

*Dr. Dale*

## THIS WEEK'S ASSIGNMENT
• Make a sign with your semester GPA goal.
•Show your sign to your accountability buddy.

# Week 15

# FIVE SIGNS YOU NEED A TUTOR

*To my premedical friend:*

If you remember nothing else from this letter, remember this: Pride always comes before the fall. Many premedical students refuse to use tutors because they think it is a sign of failure. Students who refuse to use tutors don't realize that other students who are making better grades than them are using tutors. Sometimes it is difficult to know when you need help, so here are five signs that you need a tutor.

1) **You have a B or below in the class.** Many students feel as though they should only request a tutor if they're failing a course, but this certainly is not the case. Along the premed journey, your goal is to make as many "A"s as possible. Though this is not a requirement, it should certainly be something you set out to do. It is important to realize that many colleges have free tutoring services. If you do not have an "A" in a course, why not take advantage of the service.

2) **You are spending too much time studying for a single subject.** In certain situations, even though you may be doing well in a particular class, you could be spending too much time studying for that subject. This in turn takes away from your time to study for other courses. In such cases, you should consider getting a tutor for that course because having one might decrease the time you need to spend on the material. By doing this, you free up time to study for other classes.

3) **Your professor recommends it.** This is simple enough. If your professor suggests that you get a tutor, consider it. Not only will it help you do better in the class, it will demonstrate to your professor that you are coachable and took his or her advice in hopes of performing better. If he or she writes you a recommendation letter, this will speak highly of your character.

4) **You don't have a deep understanding of the material.** Often, we can answer questions correctly, but still lack a deep understanding of the subject matter. In such situations, getting a tutor to gain depth can prove beneficial. The better you understand the material, the less time you will spend studying, and the higher grade you can achieve. Furthermore, when you enter medical school, you will have a solid foundation to build upon.

5) **You are repeating a class.** Sometimes students wait too long to get help, and before they know it, they've performed poorly in a class and have to repeat it. If this happens to you, before you take the course again, be sure to sign up for a tutor.

My challenge to you this week is to look up the various tutoring services and their associated costs.

I'd love to hear how your challenge went. Tweet me @DoctorDaleMD #PreMedMondays. I continue to pray for your success, and I look forward to our time together next Monday.

*Dr. Dale*

## THIS WEEK'S ASSIGNMENT
• Look up the various tutoring services.
• How much do they cost?

# Week 16

# FIVE WAYS TO MAXIMIZE SELF-STUDY

*To my premedical friend:*

I hope this letter finds you well. This week I want to share with you some tips to maximize your individual study time. Keep in mind that a perfect grade point average is not enough to get you into medical school. As a premedical student, you need to be efficient in your studying to free up time to excel in other areas (premed clubs, shadowing, research, etc.). Please consider these five tips, which can help you maximize your individual study time.

1) **Always read ahead.** The first thing you must understand is that your individual study time will affect your class lecture time, which in turn will affect your individual study time. It's a vicious cycle! Reading the subject matter before class is a critical step in mastering individual study. When you attend a lecture, it should not be the

first time you are hearing the information being presented. More than likely your professor has given you a course syllabus, and you should know what the lecture topic will be weeks, if not months, in advance. Make sure you have read the subject matter ahead of time so when your professor is speaking, a good amount of that information will be a review.

2) **Go to class.** This one is pretty simple, but you'd be surprised how many premeds don't go to class (unless you are one of those premeds). Consider your class time as part of your study time. If you have read in advance, and a good portion of the material is review for you, that can knock off several hours from your weekly study time for that course. Not only should you go to class, but you should take detailed notes you can easily refer to during your evening and weekend study time. Please, go to class!

3) **Review each day's lessons that night.** In order to do this, you must go to class (I have to stress that point). Every night you should go over the lectures from that day. Read over your notes, and if time allows, rewrite your notes. During my premedical years, this was one of the habits that allowed me to perform well. I literally could recite lecture notes verbatim (ask anyone who studied with me—I'm not lying). While this might not work so well for courses that require problem-solving, it works extremely well for courses such as biology, history, and psychology.

4) **Be disciplined and consistent.** Every premedical student should have a study schedule. Tips one through three above won't work unless you have a study schedule that you are disciplined enough to adhere to. Discipline

and consistency are critical keys to all success!

5) **Take study breaks.** For a long time, I didn't believe in the concept of burnout. Then I burned out. This is a real phenomenon, and you need to know how to use study breaks appropriately to prevent it. Breaks can be fifteen minutes while studying during the evening, or a full day over the course of a weekend. Besides long holidays, it is rare that you should take a study break longer than a full day. In order to have a break, by definition, you must be active in something that you can break from. Master tips one to four above so you can earn that break time!

My challenge to you this week is for you to draft a study schedule. If possible, have some overlapping time so you can take breaks with your accountability buddy.

I'd love to hear how your challenge went. Tweet me @DoctorDaleMD #PreMedMondays. I continue to pray for your success, and I look forward to our time together next Monday.

*Dr. Dale*

## THIS WEEK'S ASSIGNMENT
- Write down your upcoming study schedule.
- If possible, take breaks with your accountability buddy.

# Week 17

# BELIEVE IN YOURSELF

*To my premedical friend:*

Can I be honest with you?

There was a time in my life when I valued other people's assessment of my future as much as I did my own. If someone didn't have confidence in my abilities, it hurt my heart. I didn't realize the simple truth that, in order for me to be successful, only one person had to believe in me. That one person was me. Do you understand that about yourself?

I'm sure you know this by now, but there will be many challenges on your journey to become a medical student, and eventually a medical doctor.

You certainly will have times when you will doubt yourself, and that is okay. It is also okay for you to seek support and encouragement from others. That said, it is of extreme importance that you learn to value your own opinion pertaining to your abilities, more than you value the opinions of others. Believe in yourself! Before you ask anybody else to believe in you, you must first believe in yourself.

I hope you realize that there is no reason why you cannot become a medical doctor. We all have our own individual trials in life, and certainly more will come. In order to overcome them, we must first believe in ourselves and after that, if necessary, ask others to believe in us.

My challenge to you this week is for you to write down an affirmation, a statement of confidence demonstrating that you believe in yourself.

I'd love to hear how your challenge went. Tweet me @DoctorDaleMD #PreMedMondays. I continue to pray for your success, and I look forward to our time together next Monday.

*Dr. Dale*

## THIS WEEK'S ASSIGNMENT
• Write down your affirmation statement.
• Share your affirmation with your accountability buddy.

# Week 18

# FIVE KEYS TO MAXIMIZE GROUP STUDY TIME

*To my premedical friend:*

I hope all is well on your end. Two weeks ago, I wrote to you about making the most of your individual study time. This week, I want to discuss group study. There is plenty to be gained from studying in groups, the key is to maximize your time together and to not just socialize. Here are five tips to help you optimize your group study time:

1) **Choose your group wisely.** If you get only one thing right about group study, make sure it's this first tip. Everyone in the group must benefit from a collaborative effort focused on the goal of achieving an "A" in that course. It is okay for you all to be friends and have fun, but it is also essential that you can focus when it's time to focus. The people you choose to study with can make or break your grade, so choose wisely!

2) **Limit your group study time.** Let's be real—it is very easy for group study time to turn into social hour. One of the best ways to prevent this from happening is to limit the amount of time you spend studying together. If the group agrees beforehand to limit the study time to two hours, you are more likely to stay focused. You should also keep in mind that not everyone in your group will have the same level of understanding pertaining to each topic. Knowing this, be cognizant of the time spent catching others up. It is important to take extra time if you need to help someone, but one person should not consistently slow down the entire group. In those situations, that individual should be asked to do more self-study so he or she can contribute more to helping others.

3) **Use your group study time as a review session.** To get the most out of group study, the members of your group should not show up expecting to learn new concepts from each other. Individuals who do this will disrupt learning for others and bring down the group. Group study sessions should, for the most part, be a review. Each person in the group should come with a decent understanding of the topic at hand.

4) **Use your group study time as an opportunity to test your knowledge.** Perhaps the best thing about taking part in group study sessions is that you can use them as opportunities to test your own knowledge. The way you do this is by teaching others. Even if everyone in the group seems to understand the subject matter, take turns teaching one another and answering questions. This allows you to determine if you have a deep understanding of the material.

5) **Have a study session plan.** Never show up to a group study session without knowing exactly what you will be reviewing. That is an excellent way to waste your time. You'll end up spending the first ten minutes simply deciding what to review. Before every session, all of the group members should know what the topic of discussion will be and should have already studied it.

My challenge to you this week is to make a plan for your next group study session. In this plan, make it clear that students will be expected to teach one another.

I'd love to hear how your challenge went. Tweet me @DoctorDaleMD #PreMedMondays. I continue to pray for your success, and I look forward to our time together next Monday.

*Dr. Dale*

## THIS WEEK'S ASSIGNMENT
- Write down a plan for your next group study session.
- Which topic(s) will each student be expected to teach?

# Week 19

# FIVE WAYS TO MAXIMIZE CLASSROOM TIME

*To my premedical friend:*

In the modern age of technology, much of your learning can be done online. This has led to many students not attending class simply because they feel they can get the same information without attending. The truth is, if you understand how to maximize your classroom time, you will likely perform better overall. Here are five ways to maximize your classroom time. Note: most of these tips have been highlighted already, but these are crucial principles for success!

1) **Go to class.** You cannot maximize your classroom time if you are not there. The online video lectures and PowerPoints provided by your professors are typically meant to be supplementary (unless it's an online course). Do not rely on them to get you the grades you need. If nothing else, consider the fact that some professors give

extra credit to the students who actually attend. Your professors get up and show up for class on time, and you should do the same.

2) **Sit in the front row.** This is a constant theme throughout this book, and it cannot be overemphasized. Sitting in the front row is priceless when it comes to your success. Find that special seat and make sure your classmates know that it has your name on it.

3) **Put your cell phone on silent.** Those social media notifications can be answered later. You may feel as though you need to be available for others twenty-four hours a day, but the truth of the matter is, you do not. At the very least, you should turn off your social media alerts.

4) **Take notes.** It is easy to get in the habit of relying on PowerPoints and class scribe notes, but writing your own notes will help you retain the information. This will also keep you alert during class.

5) **Ask questions.** If you do not feel comfortable asking questions during the lecture, then stay after class for a couple of minutes. There is no sense in leaving a lecture knowing you have a question that your professor could answer in a matter of seconds. The alternative is for you to spend minutes, if not hours, trying to figure it out at home.

My challenge to you this week is to stay after one of your lectures to ask a specific question to your professor. If you have not been formally introduced, be sure to shake hands and state your full name.

I'd love to hear how your challenge went. Tweet me @DoctorDaleMD #PreMedMondays. I continue to pray for your success, and I look forward to our time together next Monday.

*Dr. Dale*

## THIS WEEK'S ASSIGNMENT

• When you stay after class to speak with your professor, what question(s) will you ask?

• With your accountability buddy, practice giving a firm handshake and stating your full name when introducing yourself to professors and future mentors.

# Week 20

# FIVE REASONS TO SIT IN THE FRONT OF THE CLASS

*To my premedical friend:*

I want to share one of the biggest premed success secrets with you. This secret proved very rewarding for me during my undergraduate years. It is the secret of the front row. Yes, I know that this is often considered to be the worst seat you can have in class. You can't fall asleep, you can't talk to your friends, and you can't text on your cell phone. And that's exactly why you want to sit in the front row.

As a premedical student, your mindset matters. You need to appreciate the fact that the front row seats are the best seats in the class. Here are five reasons you should always sit in the front row:

1) **You have fewer distractions.** When you sit in the back (or middle) of the class, you are distracted by every other student sitting in front of you. You can see who is

perusing random websites that have nothing to do with the class. Even when you are trying to listen to your professor, these distractions are hard to ignore. When you sit in the front row, all of these distractions are immediately eliminated.

2) **You will gain the confidence to interact with the professor.** It is much easier to ask a question in class when the only person you can see in front of you is your professor. When you sit in the back of the classroom, there is an automatic intimidation factor that discourages students from asking questions. When you ask a question from the back, everybody turns around to stare at you. *Is this a dumb question?* That thought will certainly go through your head. However, when you sit in the front row, you can't see who's looking at you; therefore, your confidence level increases.

3) **You will stay more alert.** An obvious reason to sit in the front row is that you are held accountable by your professor. It looks really bad if you fall asleep in the front row while the professor is standing directly in front of you. If you do, you are practically begging your professor to tease you in front of the entire classroom. Sitting in the front row will hold you accountable and encourage you to stay awake. In order to make all "A"s, you have to pay attention, and the first step in paying attention is to stay awake.

4) **Your professor will remember you.** Professors know the students who inhabit the front row. These students are typically go-getters, and when you sit there, in your professor's mind, you automatically become one of them. Also, by sitting in the front row, it is likely that you will ask more questions which will make you more

memorable to your professor. This will be important when it comes time for you to ask for recommendation letters to medical school. Start building your relationship by forming a good impression of yourself in your professor's mind.

5) **It boosts your confidence.** It is difficult to describe, but there is something special about sitting front and center. It gives you a sense of belonging and ownership in your class. Perhaps it is simply because you are more engaged, but regardless of why it happens, your confidence level will receive a boost and that will help you perform better.

My challenge to you this week is to sit in the front row of your science classes.

I'd love to see a selfie pic with you sitting there. Tweet me @DoctorDaleMD #PreMedMondays. I continue to pray for your success, and I look forward to our time together next Monday.

*Dr. Dale*

### THIS WEEK'S ASSIGNMENT
• Make it a point to arrive extra early for class so you will be sure to get a front-row seat.

*Things work out best for those who make
the best of how things work out.*

—JOHN WOODEN

# Week 21

# DISCIPLINE

*To my premedical friend:*

This week I want to discuss the concept of discipline with you. This character trait is an absolute requirement for success. If you want to join the ranks of those who call themselves physicians, you must have discipline.

Discipline is the ability to have a vision, know why it is your vision, and then carry out the tasks necessary (in a consistent manner) to accomplish that vision. It is consistently doing the right things, at the right times, for the right reasons. This is something we are taught from childhood, yet many of us drift away from its practice. I encourage you to be active in maintaining the practice of discipline.

Disciplined people tend to be very reliable and accountable. When they say they're going to do something, they do it. In reality, it is more important to keep your promises to yourself than to others because if you can't count on yourself, then there's no way others will be able to count on you. If you tell yourself you are going to read all of chapter 7 tonight, then be disciplined and read all of chapter 7 tonight. Hold yourself to a non-negotiable high standard.

People often ask me how smart you have to be to become a medical doctor. I will tell you the same thing that I tell them. It is not that you have to be smart, but rather you have to be disciplined. Nobody is born inherently smart. They become smart because they were disciplined and worked hard to achieve that. The same goes for you and me. The reason I am able to practice medicine today is because I was disciplined and held myself accountable. If you do the same, you'll be wearing your own white coat soon enough.

My challenge to you this week is to review your study schedule and evaluate how disciplined you have been in adhering to it.

I'd love to hear how your challenge went. Tweet me @DoctorDaleMD #PreMedMondays. I continue to pray for your success, and I look forward to our time together next Monday.

*Dr. Dale*

## THIS WEEK'S ASSIGNMENT
- How might you revise your study schedule to make better use of your study time? (If you do not have a study schedule, create one.)
- How disciplined have you been in following your study schedule?

# Week 22

# FIVE WAYS TO USE OFFICE HOURS WISELY

*To my premedical friend:*

Many premedical students are intimidated by the thought of going to see their professor during office hours. I remember being in your position and having that same concern. The truth of the matter is that your professors are usually excited to have students attend their office hours. The simple fact that you took time out of your day to come see them makes them do their best to accommodate your needs.

Most students don't use office hours consistently, so when you do, you become a rock star in their eyes. So, after you gather the courage to go to office hours, you need to make certain that you use that time wisely. Allow me to share five suggestions to help you get the most out of your professors' office hours or those offered by the TA's (teaching assistants).

1) **Meet with your professor one week before each test.**

This is a must if you want to get straight "A"s (or anything remotely close to that). You should meet with your professor one week before every test, and have a list of questions prepared that pertain to the upcoming exam. Sometimes, you may already know the answers to the questions, but it never hurts to get a little more clarification. If you can get in the habit of doing this, I am confident that you will perform better in your classes.

2) **Obtain career advice.** This is especially true for professors in the sciences. Most of these individuals have a sense of what it takes to get into medical school because they have advised other students pursuing this career path. Use your professors for more than just learning the subject matter of the class. They are also a valuable resource for advice pertaining to your journey to medical school.

3) **Build rapport.** In the early years of your premedical journey, it is important to keep in mind that you will need people to support you when it comes time to apply for medical school. In other words, you want to have a list of professors you can call upon to write you letters of recommendation. Your professors get to know you a little from your classes, but you really build rapport by attending their office hours. Take some time during these meetings to talk about your interests, and ask your professors about their interests. Remember, they are humans too and have lives outside of your classes.

4) **Seek job opportunities.** Many premedical students are interested in getting paid to conduct research in a science lab. Office hours are a great place to connect with your professors and express your interest in their research. Not only will this look good on your medical

school application, but you might get the opportunity to have a paying job, one that is pertinent to your future, while still in college.

5) **Say thank you.** Often, we forget how much our professors do for us. They spend countless hours doing their best to make sure we are properly taught their subject matter. Sometimes it's good to simply stop by and say thank you. This is especially true after you have completed the course, and even more true after you receive your medical school acceptance letter. Your professors are human beings too. They'll appreciate a thank-you, and they'll remember you for it.

My challenge to you this week is to set up a time to meet with at least one of your professors prior to your next test.

I'd love to hear how your challenge went. Tweet me @DoctorDaleMD #PreMedMondays. I continue to pray for your success, and I look forward to our time together next Monday.

*Dr. Dale*

## THIS WEEK'S ASSIGNMENT

- Make a list with all your professors' (or TA's) office hours.
- Before your next test, schedule a time to meet with your professor.

# Week 23

# FIVE EXTRACURRICULAR ACTIVITIES TO CONSIDER

*To my premedical friend:*

As a college student, you have a tremendous amount of free time. You have more free time than you did in high school, and more free time than you will in medical school. I will be honest with you, when my mentees tell me they are busy, it makes me chuckle. On call eighty hours a week in the ICU with an infant at home—that's busy! What I want you to understand is that you have no excuse to waste time (99 percent of college students have extra time on their hands). Medical school admissions committees are looking to see what you do with that free time. Here are five extracurricular activities for you to consider as a premedical student.

1) **Physician shadowing.** This isn't something you should think about doing; it is something you must do if you want to go to medical school. You definitely want to

shadow physicians, but shadowing other clinicians such as physician assistants (PAs) and nurse practitioners (NPs) is also great experience. And to state the obvious, shadowing is important because it helps you decide if this is the career for you.

2) **Join a premedical club.** Active participation in a premedical society provides great benefits. Specifically, it gives you access to resources that you otherwise might not have. You will also make great friends in the process.

3) **Write.** Nowadays in the digital age, more and more students are taking on blogging. This helps to improve your communication skills and allows other people to understand your thoughts. What's even better is that it helps you understand your own thoughts and allows you to clarify your stance on certain issues. Traditionally, this has not been thought of as a major premed extracurricular activity, but in the world of social media where your content can be seen anywhere, bloggers are valued more and more every day.

4) **Volunteer.** This is an obvious one. If you want to go to medical school, where the focus is to learn how to help people, you need to demonstrate now that you are doing things to help people. Volunteer opportunities are very easy to come by, especially on college campuses. Not only does this look good on your application, but more importantly, it teaches you what it truly means to serve and help others.

5) **Travel.** This is a great way to have fun and learn at the same time. Exploring the world is one of the most beneficial educational experiences a student can have. You learn that life is bigger than you think it is and there are

different ways to do things. If you can do this via some sort of study abroad, or learner exchange program, that is even better than vacation traveling.

Please use your time wisely. It is one of our greatest gifts, yet it is perhaps the one we waste the most. Medical schools will ask you to account for the time spent during your premed years. Remember that you are on a mission to care for human life. Many of your friends will not value time as much as you might, and they may encourage you to squander it. Please don't. Be wise!

My challenge to you this week is to calculate how many hours you have each week when you are awake, but not in class. How do you spend those hours?

I'd love to hear how your challenge went. Tweet me @DoctorDaleMD #PreMedMondays. I continue to pray for your success, and I look forward to our time together next Monday.

*Dr. Dale*

## THIS WEEK'S ASSIGNMENT

- Not counting class time, how many waking hours do you have?
- Write down how you will spend those hours each week.

# Week 24

# FIVE TIPS FOR A GREAT SHADOWING EXPERIENCE

*To my premedical friend:*

You need to have a good idea of what physicians do on a daily basis before you commit to this career. The most common way to get this exposure is via shadowing. Unfortunately (or fortunately for some), one bad shadowing experience can destroy a premedical student's dream of becoming a doctor. That being the case, it is of utmost importance that your shadowing experiences are excellent. Here are five tips to help you accomplish that:

1) **Shadow for two hours at a time.** Doing this will help you and the clinician remain engaged with one another for the duration of your time there. The longer you are there, the longer you distract the doctor from completing his or her work. Also, as a premedical student, even though you are passionate about medicine, a lot of the

information will fly over your head. The result of that is often boredom. Two hours is the just the right amount of time.

2) **Look the part.** When you arrive at the clinic or hospital, you don't want to stand out. Remember, the nail that sticks out gets hammered. Look the part. Even if you are a strong-willed individual determined to show your individuality, remember that while there, you represent the physician you are shadowing. It is very possible that if you are not dressed appropriately, you will be asked to leave, and that may ruin your chances of shadowing at that particular clinic or hospital again.

3) **Be a fly on the wall.** Shadowing a physician isn't like interacting with your professor in class. The doctor you are shadowing will likely be very busy. The truth is, many physicians view student shadowing as a burden to accomplishing their work. Therefore, if you are not viewed this way, they will consider it a positive experience. If possible, save your questions until the physician is taking a break or is done for the day. If the pace is rather slow, it's okay to ask questions as you go.

4) **Take notes.** I don't mean scribe the doctor's notes, but rather write down any questions that you may have. This will keep you engaged, and the physician will be able to see that you are interested. If you do not have time to ask questions at the end of the day, you can email one or two questions to the physician as a means of staying in touch.

5) **Form a relationship with the physician.** One goal of your shadowing experience should be to develop a good relationship with the physician. If you do, make sure to

seek further shadowing opportunities with him or her. When you come back next time, the physician will be more inclined to spend time teaching since he or she now has a vested interest in your learning and you are no longer a stranger to them. Additionally, this individual might be willing to write you a great letter of recommendation.

My challenge to you this week is to find a physician and set up a time to shadow during your next break.

I'd love to hear how your challenge went. Tweet me @DoctorDaleMD #PreMedMondays. I continue to pray for your success, and I look forward to our time together next Monday.

*Dr. Dale*

## THIS WEEK'S ASSIGNMENT
• Find a physician to shadow.

# Week 25

# INVEST IN YOURSELF

*To my premedical friend:*

This week I want to share something that I never understood when I was in your position. Although I did it to a certain degree, had I better understood this concept, I might have been spared from many "failures." The concept I am referring to is self-investment.

The idea of investment is very simple. You give away something of value and expect to gain something back of greater value. The process of gaining something back is called a "return on investment" (ROI).

Here's an example most premedical students will understand. Medical school is very expensive, and most students borrow loans to finance it. Often, we consider these loans as debt. Yes, it is true they are debt, but what is even more true is that they are investments. Throughout your career as a medical doctor, you will make more money than the amount of debt you would have accumulated through loans. You will also help people in ways that would otherwise not have been possible had you not taken out those loans.

Let me ask you this question: What is the difference between a rich man's mindset and a poor man's mindset? The poor man's mindset is to spend whereas the rich man's mindset is to invest. Technically, you cannot spend without investing, nor can you invest without spending. But it is the mindset that I want you to focus on.

When you study, you will be more productive if you think of that time as an investment in your success as opposed to thinking of that time as being merely spent on studying. The idea of spending implies that you will not get anything of enduring value in return. Do not ever spend your money or time. Always invest in success!

Throughout your premedical years, there will be many opportunities that arise. When deciding which opportunities to pursue, go with the ones that are good investments and avoid the ones that are simply spending. If you can master this practice, your future will certainly be bright as a medical doctor.

My challenge to you this week is to identify at least one thing that you are spending your time on instead of investing it. Decide whether this one thing is important enough that you need to continue doing it.

I'd love to hear how your challenge went. Tweet me @DoctorDaleMD #PreMedMondays. I continue to pray for your success, and I look forward to our time together next Monday.

*Dr. Dale*

**THIS WEEK'S ASSIGNMENT**
- What is one thing you are spending your time on instead of investing it?
- Is this activity important enough that you need to continue doing it?

# Week 26

# FIVE REASONS TO CONSIDER UNDERGRADUATE RESEARCH

*To my premedical friend:*

The search for knowledge is a core value of every academic institution. As a medical doctor, you will be a lifelong learner with the goal of obtaining as much knowledge as humanly possible. This God-given knowledge allows us to improve the health of our fellow humans. While it is true that research is not fitting for every premedical student, medical schools do tend to look favorably upon those who have participated in it. Here are five reasons that every premedical student should at least consider conducting research:

1) **Research provides great learning opportunities.** Typically, premedical students conduct research with science professors. This allows you to gain expertise in the specific area in which your studies are focused. For example, if you were doing research on Drosophila

melanogaster (fruit flies), you would likely gain a better understanding of genetics. No matter what area you are conducting your research in, do your best to gain extra expertise in it.

2) **You can build a strong relationship with a professor.** Conducting research is a great way to develop an excellent relationship with a professor. This professor will likely become a strong mentor for you and invest his or her time and efforts into your success. Furthermore, when it comes time for you to request letters of recommendation for medical school, assuming you did a good job, this professor will gladly write you a wonderful letter.

3) **You might get paid.** Many undergraduate students are looking for a paying job while in college. Conducting undergraduate research is a great option for part-time employment that pays decently. Not all research positions will pay, so if you are unable to get a paid position please remember that the experience is more important than the money. However, it's good to earn a little extra cash when possible.

4) **Medical schools like research.** The bottom line is that medical schools want their applicants to show dedication to a purpose. Conducting research is a simple way to demonstrate this. It shows that you are inquisitive, reliable, and interested in the sciences. Without question, research on your medical school application is a strong bonus.

5) **You just might love it.** Obviously, this is the most important of the five considerations. Many students begin research and have no idea how much they will love

it. Once they get their feet wet, they become research addicts. Giving research a shot during your premed years will also help you decide if the MD/DO–PhD route might be the way for you to go.

My challenge to you this week is to review some of your professors' profiles to learn what type of research they conduct. See if anything piques your interest.

I'd love to hear how your challenge went. Tweet me @DoctorDaleMD #PreMedMondays. I continue to pray for your success, and I look forward to our time together next Monday.

*Dr. Dale*

### THIS WEEK'S ASSIGNMENT
• What type(s) of research do your professors conduct?
• Which research project piques your interest the most?

# Week 27

# FIVE REASONS TO CONSIDER STUDYING ABROAD

*To my premedical friend:*

It's very easy to get comfortable with where you are in life. I'm referring to where you are at both physically and mentally. There's much to be gained by experiencing something different. Studying abroad is a wonderful way to do that. In full disclosure, I didn't do this, but should the opportunity arise, I certainly would. Here are five reasons to consider studying abroad:

1) **You can learn a new language.** You may not become fluent, but you'll learn enough to get by. Day by day, our world is becoming more global. No matter what field you go into, medicine included, being familiar with multiple languages is beneficial.

2) **You will get exposure to a different culture.** While learning a new language is part of experiencing a cul-

ture, there's much more to it than that. The way people dress, the foods they eat, the way they greet one another, the intent behind their actions—all of these things are a part of a society's culture. It is important to gain an understanding of how other people function in the world, and to acknowledge that there are other ways to live besides the way you do.

3) **You will make new friends.** It is important to remember that life continues, even while you are on the pre-med journey. Friends are important, and they are part of your journey. Studying abroad will give you the opportunity to make brand-new friends who you would have never met otherwise. These can become lifelong friendships.

4) **You will gain an appreciation of your own culture.** You have probably heard the saying, "You don't know what you've got until it's gone." Well, even though your culture won't be gone when you are studying abroad, just being away can give you a greater appreciation. Simple conveniences that you take for granted every day will be brought to light when overseas. Such things will give you a greater appreciation for your homeland.

5) **It's just a really cool thing to do.** Not too many people can say they have traveled to a foreign country and spent several months there. When you look back at this later in your life, it'll be a really cool thing to tell people. That in and of itself is enough!

My challenge to you this week is to spend five minutes talking to someone from a different country. Step outside of your box and learn to appreciate someone different.

I'd love to hear how your challenge went. Tweet me

@DoctorDaleMD #PreMedMondays. I continue to pray for your success, and I look forward to our time together next Monday.

*Dr. Dale*

**THIS WEEK'S ASSIGNMENT**
• Take five minutes to talk to someone from a different country.
• How did you learn to better appreciate that person?

# Week 28

# FIVE MEDICALLY RELATED JOBS FOR PREMEDS

*To my premedical friend:*

When it comes to job opportunities, premeds have it nice. There are many jobs out there that will not only pay you, but also give you phenomenal exposure to the medical field. It should go without saying that if your grades are not up to par, and you do not have to work to support yourself or your family, then you should focus on your education before getting a job. For those of you who can work, here are five medically related jobs to consider:

1) **Medical scribe.** Medical scribes take notes for clinicians during patient encounters. This job puts you directly in the mix of things. Not only do you get to see all the action, but you also get to document the action in the actual note that will end up in that patient's medical records. It's hard to beat this experience.

2) **Phlebotomist**. A phlebotomist is an individual who draws blood from patients. It should go without saying that a requirement for this job is your ability to tolerate the sight of blood. This job not only puts you in the clinical environment, but it gives you real hands-on experience with patients.

3) **A nurse technician.** These individuals work closely with nurses to provide frontline care for patients. From checking vital signs to bathing patients, you are definitely in the mix. An added advantage to this job is once you become a physician, you'll have a better appreciation for the work nurses do.

4) **A bedside attendant, also known as a sitter.** There are plenty of patients in the hospital who cannot be alone in their rooms. These individuals often need redirection to keep them safe from harming themselves, or need assistance when they want to contact their healthcare providers. The main job of a bedside attendant is to monitor for the patient's safety and call for help when the patient cannot. This is also a good job to have if you'd like to get some studying done while at work.

5) **A blogger.** This one is a little bit different. While you are not physically involved in patient care, you are intellectually engaged in the field of medicine. Writing blogs is also great because you can typically do it when you want, and from where you want. Furthermore, in this day and age of social media, more and more doctors are interested in medical journalism. This would be a great start. I must caution, however, that it is difficult to get paid for writing blogs in the premedical world. The reality of the situation is that many students like to write and blog simply to express their opinions.

My challenge to you this week is to search for medically related jobs in your area. Are any of them a good fit for you? Discuss these jobs with your accountability buddy.

I'd love to hear how your challenge went. Tweet me @DoctorDaleMD #PreMedMondays. I continue to pray for your success, and I look forward to our time together next Monday.

*Dr. Dale*

## THIS WEEK'S ASSIGNMENT
- Make a list of medically related job openings in your area.
- Are any of them a good fit for you?
- Discuss these job opportunities with your accountability buddy.

# Week 29

# THE PREMED G.R.I.N.D.

*To my premedical friend:*

Anybody who knows me knows the value I place on hard work. I am a firm believer that if you want something in life, you should never expect someone to give it to you, and you should grind to get it. Grind. It's such an excellent word, isn't it? As a matter of fact, it's one of my favorites. When I'm invited to speak at various events, you'll often hear me use it somewhere in my presentation. There's just something about that word that carries an immense amount of power. But my question to you is, Do you grind? If so how? Let me tell you how I G.R.I.N.D.

**G stands Goals.** I set a lot of these and write them down so I can't run away from them. On the very laptop that I am using to write this book, I have a document containing my goals. The first step in accomplishing something is to have something to accomplish. Set your goals, write them down, and tell a friend. As a premed, a simple goal might be to get a higher GPA than the average medical school student. Or you may set a goal to acquire twenty shadowing hours this summer.

**R stands for Resolve.** This is where the power of positive thinking comes in to play. There is absolutely no point in setting goals if you don't resolve to achieve them. You must believe in yourself and commit to resilience. You'll get knocked down multiple times along the way, but once you resolved to make it happen, only you can choose to stop.

**I stands for Information.** We live in an age of information. Never before have we had such easy access to knowledge. The old excuse, "I didn't know" doesn't work anymore. Once you set your goal and resolve to accomplish it, you need to gather the necessary information to make it happen. So, you want to publish a research paper? Well, do you know how to conduct the research? Do you know what journal to submit your manuscript to? Get the knowledge.

**N stands for Network.** Nothing great happens without a team effort. Michael Jordan didn't win a championship, the Chicago Bulls organization did. Show me your five best friends, and I'll tell you how successful you'll be. To accomplish your goals, you must have people in your network that can help you along the way. You want to be a doctor? Are you surrounded by doctors, or future doctors? You'll only go as far as your network takes you.

**D stands for Discipline.** *Goals, Resolve, Information,* and *Network.* None of these mean a thing if you aren't disciplined enough to do what you are supposed to do. Premedical students often ask me how they can know if they are smart enough to become a doctor. My response is typically, "That's the wrong question to ask." Most of us are smart enough, so the real question is, Are you disciplined enough? The greatest in life are the most disciplined.

This is how I G.R.I.N.D. every day. It is my basic approach to success, which I am now sharing with you and I pray you implement in your life. I've chatted with enough of the PreMed STAR students to understand your doubts and frustrations about the premedical journey. It's a tough road that can get really ugly along the way. But just know that you've got a strong network of future doctors alongside you. Support one another. Share resources, ask questions, and do it together. Through this premed G.R.I.N.D., you'll become a better person, and in the end, there will be a white coat with your name on it.

My challenge to you this week is to memorize G.R.I.N.D. and discuss it with your accountability buddy.

I'd love to hear how your challenge went. Tweet me @DoctorDaleMD #PreMedMondays. I continue to pray for your success, and I look forward to our time together next Monday.

*Dr. Dale*

## THIS WEEK'S ASSIGNMENT
• What do each of these mean to you?
- Goals
- Resolve
- Information
- Network
- Discipline
• Tell your accountability buddy how you plan to G.R.I.N.D. this week.

# Week 30

# FIVE WAYS TO SPEND YOUR SUMMERS

*To my premedical friend:*

Your summers are extremely valuable. They are opportunities to enrich yourself and enhance your curriculum vitae. Unless it is absolutely necessary (e.g., family emergencies), no premedical student should spend the summer doing anything that will not encourage him or her to pursue a career in medicine. Here are five excellent ways to spend your summer:

1) **Shadow a physician.** If you want to be a medical doctor, you have to know what it's like to be a medical doctor. One of the best ways to do that is by shadowing clinicians, and one of the best times to do it is during your summer vacation. Not only will this expose you to medicine, but it's also an opportunity to gain a mentor.

2) **Summer school.** When we think about summer school, we tend to think about having to repeat courses. Yes,

sometimes this is the case, but many people also use summers to get ahead in their classes. This in turn can lighten the load for future semesters. Also keep in mind that many students take some of the more challenging premed courses in the summer. This is okay, but do know that some medical school admission committee members frown upon this. In their mind, students do this to avoid the challenge of taking a tough class with a heavier course load.

3) **Summer enrichment programs.** There are many summer enrichment programs across the country. Most are held at academic medical centers, but some can be found in community hospitals as well. These programs typically provide a nice variety of experiences to broaden your exposure. Another perk of these programs is they may come with a stipend.

4) **Study abroad.** Summer is the perfect time to get away and experience the world. You can use this time to take courses, but being in a different country is enriching in itself. The exposure to different cultures will mold you into a more well-rounded individual and medical school candidate.

5) **Research internship.** Conducting research during the summer is a great way to get your feet wet. The projects are often short and clearly planned ahead of time because the mentors know you are only there for few weeks. Also, for students who are uncertain about if research is right for them, this is a great way to test it out. Not to mention, many summer research programs pay rather well.

My challenge to you this week is to make a list of ten

summer opportunities you are interested in. It's important to know that the application process for many summer programs begins in the fall semester. Therefore, you must plan relatively early in the academic year.

I'd love to hear how your challenge went. Tweet me @DoctorDaleMD #PreMedMondays. I continue to pray for your success, and I look forward to our time together next Monday.

*Dr. Dale*

## THIS WEEK'S ASSIGNMENT

- Make a list of ten summer opportunities you are interested in.

   1)
   2)
   3)
   4)
   5)
   6)
   7)
   8)
   9)
   10)

- When do you need to start applying to the programs above?

*Try not to become a person of success,*
*but rather try to become a person of value.*

—ALBERT EINSTEIN

# Week 31

# FIVE TIPS TO CREATE AN AMAZING CURRICULUM VITAE

*To my premedical friend:*

I have two questions for you. First, is your curriculum vitae (CV) up to date? As a rule of thumb, this should always be the case because you never know when someone will ask for it. Second, do you have a well-written CV? It's one thing to have it prepared—it's another thing to make sure it's up to par. Here are five tips to help you put together a great curriculum vitae:

1) **Be certain there are no errors.** A quick way to get yourself thrown out of the competition is for your evaluator to find a spelling or grammatical error in your CV. If you haven't taken the necessary time to proofread it in detail, then you won't spend the necessary time to do a good job in the position they are considering you for.

2) **Choose your email wisely.** It is a good idea to use an email that contains your name. At minimum, this email

should contain either your first or last name. You certainly do not want the evaluator of your CV to send an email to baddestchick@fakeemail.com. That's another quick way to get your application tossed out.

3) **Emphasize the things that you have accomplished.** The purpose of your CV is to show people that you are capable of accomplishing things. It is important to not merely list tasks you have done, but rather focus on what you've actually accomplished. For example, don't just write that you were the president of your premed club; also add the things you did as president.

4) **Make it aesthetically pleasing.** When someone picks up your CV, it should be reader-friendly. The format needs to be easy to follow, and the font should be simple and pleasing to the eye.

5) **Start with your credentials.** In the world of academia, credentials matter. Be sure to list your academic institution and any degrees you might have near the beginning of your CV. Don't send people on wild goose chases to determine if you even have the academic credentials for the position. Your degrees, certificates, and licenses should be among the first things listed.

My challenge to you this week is to update your PreMed STAR profile (which is a CV). Review your accountability buddy's profile and ask him or her to do the same for you. What improvements did you make after doing this?

I'd love to hear how your challenge went. Tweet me @DoctorDaleMD #PreMedMondays. I continue to pray for your success, and I look forward to our time together next Monday.

*Dr. Dale*

## THIS WEEK'S ASSIGNMENT

- With your accountability buddy's input, review your PreMed STAR profile.
- What kind of updates should you make?

# Week 32

# FIVE MUST-KNOW DATES

*To my premedical friend:*

In life, always remember the low-hanging fruit. One of the easiest ways to not get accepted to medical school is to miss a deadline. As a premedical student, there are key dates that you must know or else you'll blow your chance. Here are five of them:

1) **The MCAT.** The MCAT is offered multiple times a year so you have options as to when you will take it. You need to pick the perfect MCAT date that will give adequate time to study and submit your medical school application.

2) **Medical school application opening date.** The three application services to be aware of are AMCAS, AACOMAS, and TMDSAS. It is important to maximize the time you have between the opening of applications and the first day applications can be submitted. You want to use every available minute to perfect the appli-

cation you will be submitting. Last week, I challenged you to update you PreMed STAR profile. If you keep it updated, completing your medical school applications in due time will be much easier.

3) **First day to submit medical school applications.** In ideal circumstances, you want to submit your application as soon as possible. This is important because some medical schools admit students on a rolling admissions basis. The earlier you get your application submitted, the more time admissions committees have to review it. As the cycle progresses, more and more students are submitting applications, which in turn makes the medical school admission committees very busy. Yes, I am encouraging you to submit your application early, but also make sure it's flawless.

4) **Early decision program deadline.** This program offered by medical schools through AAMC allows premedical students to confirm acceptance to medical school by a certain date every year. There are some limitations to your application process if you choose to go this route, so you will want to investigate this option in detail.

5) **Application submission deadlines.** Each individual medical school sets its own application deadlines. It is important that you know which medical schools you are interested in, and that you look up their deadlines in advance. Hopefully, you will be submitting your application relatively early and deadlines will not be an issue.

My challenge to you this week is to look up the various opening dates for the medical school application services. Add these dates to your calendar to make sure you stay on top of things!

I'd love to hear how your challenge went. Tweet me @DoctorDaleMD #PreMedMondays. I continue to pray for your success, and I look forward to our time together next Monday.

*Dr. Dale*

## THIS WEEK'S ASSIGNMENT
- Look up the various opening dates for the medical school application services.
- Add these dates to your calendar.

# Week 33

# GIFTS AND WORK

*To my premedical friend:*

Do you know the difference between your work and your job? Most people don't. As a matter of fact, most people would say that they are one in the same. That isn't the case at all, and I want you to have a clear understanding of this. It will prove useful as you fight your way through your premedical years.

A job is something you do primarily for sustainability. You provide a service of value to someone, and in return they give you something of value, typically money. Your job is external to you. You have to go out to find it then negotiate terms. Most of us aren't in control of our jobs. Jobs are temporary, and they come and go. If you are not performing well, you can be fired.

Work, on the other hand, pertains to your destiny and self-fulfillment. Unlike a job, which is about the things you do, work is about who you become. All of us are gifted by God with specific talents that we are to identify, develop, then use to benefit others. These gifts are meant to be used for our work. They cannot be taken away from us nor can we lose them. We can, however, neglect them and miss out on all the wonderful things that come with them.

This is a difficult concept, so I will use myself as an example. Before I do that, let me ask you two questions to get you in the proper frame of mind. First question: What are you good at? Second question: What things in life seem to come more natural to you than they do to others? When you can answer these two things, becoming aware of your gifts, and from that your work, will be much easier.

I am most gifted in three areas: vision, understanding, and development. These have been identified in me by others since I was a child; however, it's not until I became an adult that I came to appreciate and utilize them. They have proven extremely useful for my roles as a physician and entrepreneur. I have used these gifts to take care of some of the sickest patients in the world (I am an ICU doctor) as well as to start a couple of companies focused on developing people. Now I am using them to write you these letters.

I want you to understand that your work is more important than your job. What are you called to do during your time on earth? What gifts has God given you to accomplish these tasks? As you travel this premedical path, please keep this letter in mind.

Find your gifts! Strengthen them! Know your work and make sure your job is aligned with it.

This is a difficult concept for people to grasp. I struggled with it myself for years, but once I came to an understanding, a weight was lifted off my shoulder. I am so excited for you to find your gifts and work.

My challenge to you this week is to discuss this concept of work versus job with your accountability buddy.

I'd love to hear how your challenge went. Tweet me @DoctorDaleMD #PreMedMondays. I continue to pray for your success, and I look forward to our time together next Monday.

*Dr. Dale*

## THIS WEEK'S ASSIGNMENT
• What are your gifts (i.e. God-given talents)? We all have some. Discuss them with your accountability buddy.

# Week 34

# FIVE TIPS FOR GETTING GREAT LETTERS OF RECOMMENDATION

*To my premedical friend:*

Whether we like it or not, what others think about us matters. Medical schools understand this, which is why they ask for recommendation letters. The thing to know about your recommendation letters is that you don't want them to be good. Instead, you need them to be great! Here are five tips to get great recommendation letters:

1) **Ask for a great letter of recommendation.** This is the simplest of the five, yet it is the most powerful. Simply asking the person who writes your letter if they can write a great letter for you, will put you a step ahead of everybody else. This is a tough question to ask, so be prepared for a tough answer. Sometimes your question might be answered with a no. If this is the case, consider finding someone else to write your letter. The take-away here is

that when asking for a letter, it is important to use qualifying words such as great, exceptional, phenomenal, or outstanding.

2) **Ask the right individuals.** Premedical students often want to ask the big-name professor on campus to write a recommendation letter. What you need to understand is that big-name professors will have numerous students asking for a letter. They might end up being too busy to submit the letter within a reasonable time. Furthermore, because they might be so busy, they might not spend adequate time to write you the "great" letter you asked for. The key here is to ask individuals who know you well. If that happens to be the big name on campus, then great, but if not, stick with that individual. It is much better to get a personal letter that really speaks of who you are as a person than to get a generic letter submitted in support of your application.

3) **Ask early.** Be sure to ask your potential letter writers at least six months prior to when you expect to submit your medical school applications. Asking early will put you first in line and give your writers more time to focus on your letter. You don't want to get caught up in the rush with everyone else.

4) **Provide your letter writers with your curriculum vitae.** Although they may know you from class, the research lab, or clinic, they won't know everything about you. Providing them your premedical activities and accomplishments is essential. It's also easy to do. You can use your PreMed STAR profile to keep track of all these things, and when it's time to ask for your letter, simply email it to them.

5) **Provide them with a draft of your personal statement.**
Similar to providing your letter writers with your portfolio, giving them your personal statement will allow them to get a better understanding of who you are as an individual. Your personal statement will speak of your character and your "why." Having this information makes it much easier for a letter writer to create the great recommendation you asked for. (For more info on writing a great personal statement, see week 38.)

My challenge to you this week is to send an "update email" to two people you think would be great letter writers. Let them know how things are going for you and tell them you just wanted to keep in touch.

I'd love to hear how your challenge went. Tweet me @DoctorDaleMD #PreMedMondays. I continue to pray for your success, and I look forward to our time together next Monday.

*Dr. Dale*

**THIS WEEK'S ASSIGNMENT**
• Who could write great letters of recommendation for you?
• Send an "update email" to two of them this week.

# Week 35

# FIVE THINGS TO KNOW ABOUT THE MCAT

*To my premedical friend:*

It is believed by many that the Medical College Admissions Test (a.k.a. MCAT) is the most difficult test you will take during your premedical years. In fact, it can be argued that it is the most important test of your entire career. Since this test is so crucial to your success, you should have an excellent understanding of it. Here are five things to know about the MCAT.

1) **It's not just hard—it's very hard!** This goes without saying, especially since we just introduced the MCAT as potentially the most difficult test of your career. However, I am reiterating the level of difficulty to make sure I encourage you to over prepare rather than under prepare. Think about the hardest test you have taken in college, then multiply that difficulty by a factor of ten. That's the MCAT! Okay, I'm exaggerating a little bit. Just

know that you need to bring your "A" game.

2) **It's very long.** The MCAT is a workday's worth of testing. It's bad enough that the test is difficult, but what makes it worse is that it's also long. What this means for you is that practice MCAT tests are essential to build up your endurance.

3) **It's expensive.** Cost is important to emphasize because some premedical students assume that this test is free. This exam costs a few hundred dollars. At the time of writing this book, the MCAT cost $310. So, when planning your budget, be sure to keep this in mind.

4) **It's a deal breaker.** Unfortunately, it is true: The MCAT can make or break your dream to become a medical doctor. Although medical schools are attempting to move toward a more holistic review of the applicants, at the end of the day, numbers matter. If you perform extremely poorly on the MCAT, gaining admission to medical school will be difficult, regardless of how many Olympic gold medals you have. If you did perform below your goal, keep in mind that you can do better next time. Just refocus and attack it again!

5) **It'll be over before you know it.** Don't believe me? Just ask any doctor. You'll be surprised as you learn many of them don't even remember their MCAT score. You spend so much time and effort preparing for this exam, then the day comes, and the day goes. Work hard to get the score you need, and keep in mind, it'll be over before you know it!

My challenge to you this week is to spend some time researching the various MCAT resources. With so many to choose from, you want to have your game plan ready ahead of time! Find the ones that are right for you.

I'd love to hear how your challenge went. Tweet me @DoctorDaleMD #PreMedMondays. I continue to pray for your success, and I look forward to our time together next Monday.

*Dr. Dale*

**THIS WEEK'S ASSIGNMENT**
• Begin researching various MCAT resources.
• Which ones are right for you?

# Week 36

# FIVE THINGS TO CONSIDER WHEN PREPARING TO STUDY FOR THE MCAT

*To my premedical friend:*

As we discussed last week, the MCAT is a very important test. You must approach this test with respect and take the necessary time to develop your plan of attack. Here are five things to consider when preparing for the MCAT:

1) **Your time.** If you want to perform well on the MCAT, you will need to invest a significant amount of your time. Keep this in mind when scheduling a test date. You should give yourself at least five solid months to study for this exam. During the first four months, it would be wise to dedicate a minimum of four hours per day to MCAT studying, then ramp up to a minimum of six hours per day for at least one month. Every person is

different with regards to the exact amount of study time needed. This example is just to emphasize that a lot of time is needed.

2) **Your learning style.** Throughout your undergraduate years, you develop a certain way of studying and learning. Be mindful of this so you know the best way to get your desired grades. When the time comes to study for the MCAT, be sure to use resources that teach in ways most conducive to your learning style. For example, some people learn best by reading a textbook from cover to cover. Others learn better by watching videos. Know how you learn best, and obtain those types of resources to help you study for the MCAT.

3) **Your need for a prep course.** Do you need a test prep course? They can be extremely expensive. But if used properly, they are an investment. The truth of the matter is, they can significantly improve your scores. However, not every student needs to take a test prep. Some students are capable of performing well with self and group study. Also, when deciding if you should take a test prep course, be sure you know the teaching method the company uses. For example, how many teachers will you have? Will they use videos? How do they analyze your practice tests? These are all things for you to investigate ahead of time.

4) **Your baseline practice score.** This is perhaps the most important thing I tell my mentees pertaining to MCAT studying. You need to know your baseline score before you delve deep into studying. This is beneficial in multiple ways, including helping you to decide if you should pay for a prep course. Additionally, taking a practice exam before you start studying will help you identify

areas of weakness to focus on.

5) **Your physical and mental well-being.** This is a recurring theme for premedical students. It is very easy to get lost in the premed lifestyle of studying and staying active in various organizations. It is imperative that you remember to take care of yyourself during these stressful times. Get enough sleep, eat right, and exercise.

My challenge to you this week is to look up the average MCAT scores for three schools you are interested in.

I'd love to hear how your challenge went. Tweet me @DoctorDaleMD #PreMedMondays. I continue to pray for your success, and I look forward to our time together next Monday.

*Dr. Dale*

### THIS WEEK'S ASSIGNMENT
• What are the average MCAT scores for some of the medical schools you may be interested in attending?
• What will it take to achieve them?
• Discuss your answers with your accountability buddy.

# Week 37

# NETWORKING

*To my premedical friend:*

I am writing to you this week to discuss something I feel most premedical students are not very good at: networking. The takeaway of this letter is that things are more likely to work in your favor when you have a strong network.

I firmly believe that the success of any individual, or group, will ultimately be as strong as their network. The fact of the matter is you can't know or do everything. When the right people come together with a common goal, they can go much farther than one person going at it alone.

It is very easy for a premedical student to become isolated in their own silo. You are trained to study all day and to compete against your friends. This can lead to the toxic mentality of individualism, which is characterized by a lack of cooperation and hoarding of resources. Subsequently, your ability to network will be diminished.

While competition is a good thing, cooperation is even better. I encourage you to find a strong group of premedical students to share resources with. I am confident that if the sharing is reciprocated, you will do better with them than you will without them.

From a practical standpoint, networking will open a tremendous number of doors. Something as simple as connecting with a medical school recruiter can be the key to getting an interview at a particular school, which in turn can lead to your admission.

When you become a doctor, you will use your network every day in order to provide the best care for your patients. As a pulmonary and critical care physician (i.e., lung and ICU doctor), the deathly ill patients I care for on a daily basis depend on a strong team of physicians to help keep them alive. Networking is absolutely essential to success.

My challenge to you this week is to add at least one person to your premedical network. Don't just friend them on Facebook; make sure to add their contact information to your cell phone and connect with them on PreMed STAR.

I'd love to hear how your challenge went. Tweet me @DoctorDaleMD #PreMedMondays. I continue to pray for your success, and I look forward to our time together next Monday.

*Dr. Dale*

## THIS WEEK'S ASSIGNMENT
• Who can you add to your premedical network?
• Add their contact info to your cell phone and connect with them on PreMed STAR.

# Week 38

# FIVE TIPS FOR WRITING A GREAT PERSONAL STATEMENT

*To my premedical friend:*

Other than your medical school interview, your best shot at letting medical schools know who you really are will be your personal statement. Your personal statement will paint a picture of your dedication, passion, and commitment not only to the field of medicine, but also to the things you love. It is important that you convey this information in a concise, yet powerful way. Here are five tips for writing a great personal statement:

1) **Make it personal.** It is called a personal statement for a reason. Medical schools want to get to know you. Don't write in generic terms or use too many clichés. It is okay for you to show your heart in this essay. The reader will appreciate it.

2) **Do not embellish.** One of the worst things you can do

when writing your personal statement is to exaggerate how great of a candidate you are. Always tell the story like it is. Don't embellish even the slightest bit. If you are fortunate enough to be granted an interview, the truth will come out eventually.

3) **Write when you feel like writing.** Writer's block is a real thing, and if you wait for it to disappear, you may never get started on your personal statement. When the ideas come, you need to capture them immediately, or they might be lost forever. Even if it means getting out of bed at three o'clock in the morning, when that idea comes to you, start writing!

4). **Don't turn your personal statement into a curriculum vitae.** This is a common mistake that many premedical students make. In their eagerness to demonstrate their strengths, they list their accolades in essay format. That's what your curriculum vitae is for, not your personal statement. It's appropriate to list one or two major accomplishments, but they must contribute to the image you are painting of yourself in the white coat.

5) **Have a minimum of five people review your personal statement.** Getting feedback is extremely important. Make sure other people understand the message you are trying to convey. They need to feel your passion for medicine through the words on the paper. Aim to have at least five people proofread your essay prior to submission. Here's a word to the wise: Before you ask doctors or highly respected mentors to read your personal statement, make sure someone reviews your spelling and grammar. As someone who reads a few personal statements each year, I can tell you that an easy way to frustrate your mentor is to have them read over an essay

with numerous grammatical errors. It hinders our ability to grasp your message.

My challenge to you this week is to find a few medical school personal statements online, then proofread them. What made them good? What made them bad?

I'd love to hear how your challenge went. Tweet me @DoctorDaleMD #PreMedMondays. I continue to pray for your success, and I look forward to our time together next Monday.

*Dr. Dale*

## THIS WEEK'S ASSIGNMENT

• Find a few medical school personal statements online and proofread them.
• What made them good? What made them bad?

# Week 39

# FIVE WAYS TO GET RECRUITED TO MEDICAL SCHOOL

*To my premedical friend:*

Your chance of gaining admission into any medical school is better if their recruiters are familiar with you before they see your application. Just like with sports, the star players are the ones who get recruited, and you want to be on that list. Here are five ways to get recruited to medical school:

1) **Create a PreMed STAR profile.** It's free. PreMed STAR was built after the realization that so many qualified premeds weren't getting into medical school simply because they didn't know where to apply. For example, a student living in Florida might have no idea that a school in Michigan would love to have her. Now, students from across the country create PreMed STAR profiles and can be recruited 24/7 year round. This online recruitment network is a simple and amazing way to market yourself

to medical schools. Beyond that, PreMed STAR has tons of free resources to help you succeed.

2) **Attend events at a medical school you are interested in.** For example, if your undergraduate campus is attached to a medical school, why not go to some of their medical school events? This is a good way to interact with students and faculty. By doing this, you begin to form relationships, and the right people get to know you. When your application hits their desk, they'll remember your name and face.

3) **Volunteer or shadow at a medical school hospital.** Similar to the point above, this allows you to connect with individuals at that medical school. The concept is quite simple: The more they see you, the more they remember you.

4) **Present your research at scientific conferences.** Not only will this let you get out and meet individuals from various medical schools, but it will show them that you are a dedicated researcher who was able to present work on a higher level. This will immediately give you an upper hand. Make sure to exchange contact information with every medical school representative you meet.

5) **Attend recruitment fairs.** There are many recruitment fairs across the country. Some cost money, while others are free. There's nothing quite like shaking the hand of a med school representative and expressing your interest in their school. Whenever possible, get out there and meet some recruiters.

My challenge to you this week is to find at least one recruitment fair you can attend within the next six months.

I'd love to hear how your challenge went. Tweet me

@DoctorDaleMD #PreMedMondays. I continue to pray for your success, and I look forward to our time together next Monday.

*Dr. Dale*

**THIS WEEK'S ASSIGNMENT**
• Find at least one upcoming medical school event that you can attend.

# Week 40

# FIVE THINGS TO CONSIDER WHEN DECIDING WHICH MEDICAL SCHOOLS TO APPLY TO

*To my premedical friend:*

Applying to medical school can be a stressful process. Before you start the application process, you have to figure out which schools you'll be applying to. Nowadays, many students are applying to more than fifteen medical schools. Wow, that's a lot! But how do you know if you should apply to so many, and which ones should you apply to? Here are five things to consider:

1) **Which schools have already shown interest in you?** Your goal is to become a doctor, so you shouldn't be too proud to consider a school that has shown interest in you, no matter where that school falls on your list. Refer to last week's letter as a refresher on how you can get

recruited to medical school.

2) **Which schools are well regarded in your specific field of interest?** Most premeds aren't certain which medical specialty they will pursue, but this is important for those of you who know. If you know you want to be a cardiologist, then consider schools that have strong cardiology programs. If you go to a medical school that is reputable in the field of your interest, you have more time to form relationships with those experts, and you increase your likelihood of earning a residency position there.

3) **USMLE and COMLEX pass rates.** These are standardized exams that medical students take. The USMLE is for allopathic medical schools, and the COMLEX is for osteopathic schools. Think of these tests like the MCAT, but for medical students. You want to go to a school that has a very high pass rate. Granted, most students in the United States pass these tests, but you don't want to risk training at a school that won't prepare you well.

4) **The numbers: MCAT score and GPA.** As mentioned in a prior letter, numbers do matter. Pay attention to the average GPA of the medical schools you are applying to. This will give you an idea of how competitive you are for each individual school. Also review their websites to see if they comment on GPA requirements. Most schools will not list a hard and fast cutoff value, but some do have phrases which elude to their cutoffs. You should also keep in mind that when looking at average GPAs, some students attending that school scored lower than that average.

It's the same story for the MCAT. However, many medical schools weigh GPA more heavily than they do the

MCAT. This means that even if your MCAT is not up to par with the average for that particular school, you should still consider applying if your GPA is strong. Of course, this assumes that you have an overall strong application.

5) **Location.** Yes, your goal is to get into medical school, but if possible, why not choose a location you'll enjoy? You want to be where you are comfortable. Answer these questions: Do I want to be near friends and family? Can I tolerate the weather? How high is the cost of living? Am I okay with the major modes of transportation? These are all important to consider. Enjoying your environment will certainly help you perform better in medical school.

My challenge to you this week is to make a list of ten medical schools you will consider applying to. What specific things do you like most about your number one choice?

I'd love to hear how your challenge went. Tweet me @DoctorDaleMD #PreMedMondays. I continue to pray for your success, and I look forward to our time together next Monday.

*Dr. Dale*

## THIS WEEK'S ASSIGNMENT

• Make a list of ten medical schools you will consider applying to.

1.
2.
3.
4.
5.

6.

7.

8.

9.

10.

- What specific things do you like most about your number one choice?

*The starting point of all achievement is desire.*

—NAPOLEON HILL

# Week 41

# OUTLAST FAILURE

*To my premedical friend:*

I know you desire to be great. I know this is true because you are reading this letter. Also, if it were not, you wouldn't be pursuing one of the most challenging careers. Those of us who desire to achieve a certain level of greatness will face failure at one point or another. Some more than others. I'd like you to understand this one thing: Our biggest failures often lead to our greatest successes.

Great people don't recognize failure. Rather, they acknowledge temporary setbacks, which ultimately prove to be lessons in success. Consider all the great athletes of our day and age. Every single one has had some level of what others would consider failure, but they are great because they recognized those instances as opportunities to grow. Keep in mind that even Michael Jordan was cut from his high school varsity team.

Behind every dark cloud, there's a silver lining. This old adage has gotten me through many difficult times, because it reminds me that after the rain, the sun will shine again. What

I'm trying to tell you is that you must remain patient and out-last the rain. Success doesn't come overnight; it's an absolute grind! But if you can persevere, greatness will be there to welcome you with open arms.

My challenge to you this week is to have a discussion with your accountability buddy about something that you previously considered a failure. Discuss how that perceived failure was merely a temporary lesson and how it brought you one step closer to your vision.

I'd love to hear how your challenge went. Tweet me @DoctorDaleMD #PreMedMondays. I continue to pray for your success, and I look forward to our time together next Monday.

*Dr. Dale*

## THIS WEEK'S ASSIGNMENT
- What is a success that you previously considered a failure? Discuss this with your accountability buddy.
- Also share how that "failure" eventually brought you one step closer to your vision.

# Week 42

# FIVE DUAL-DEGREE PROGRAMS TO CONSIDER

*To my premedical friend:*

More and more physicians are looking to do other things besides practice medicine. For example, I love medicine, but I am also an entrepreneur and an author. Nowadays, many of us are more than doctors. The great thing is that medical schools are making this easier for physicians to accomplish by offering dual-degree programs. Here are five to consider:

1) **MD/DO–PhD.** This is the best-known dual-degree program. These programs focus on training physician-scientists, meaning you'll be a medical doctor who can conduct research (usually on the basic science level). Something to consider is that many of these programs pay your tuition and give you an additional stipend for living expenses. Typically, these programs take at least seven years to complete.

2) **MD/DO–MPH.** MPH stands for master in public health. Many individuals who go this route are interested in public health issues and the epidemiology of various diseases. Such individuals might want to conduct public health research, while others are looking to impact public policy and work in state health departments. This dual-degree program typically takes five to six years to complete.

3) **MD/DO–MBA.** MBA stands for master of business administration. As technology advances, the business of medicine is becoming more complicated. Society is looking for medically trained businessmen and women who understand the intricacies of healthcare delivery in resource-limited environments. Having an MBA to back your medical degree can open doors of opportunity for you. This dual-degree program typically takes five to six years to complete.

4) **MD/DO–MHA.** MHA stands for master of health administration or master of healthcare administration. The rationale for getting an MHA is somewhat similar to that of an MBA. The key difference, however, is that MHA programs typically focus more on healthcare delivery, whereas MBAs will give you a more robust understanding of business. These dual-degree programs typically take four to five years to complete.

5) **MD/DO–JD.** JD stands for Juris Doctor (doctor of law). Many individuals who pursue this career path are interested in health law, health policy, or biotechnology. These programs typically take six to seven years to complete.

My challenge to you this week is to look up one of these

dual-degree programs and find the profile of a physician with one those degrees. Try to get a sense of what that individual does for a living and if you could see yourself doing the same thing.

I'd love to hear how your challenge went. Do any of these dual-degree programs interest you? Tweet me @DoctorDaleMD #PreMedMondays. I continue to pray for your success, and I look forward to our time together next Monday.

*Dr. Dale*

---

### THIS WEEK'S ASSIGNMENT

- Of the five dual-degree programs just discussed, which one seems the most interesting?
- Find the profile of a physician with one of those degrees.
- Generally speaking, what does that individual do for a living?
- Could you see yourself doing the same thing?

# Week 43

# FIVE THINGS TO DO IN PREPARATION FOR INTERVIEW DAY

*To my premedical friend:*

Getting invited for an interview is a major accomplishment. This means the medical school sees potential in you. You've passed the paper screen, and now they want to see who you are as a real person. Your job is to shine! Here are five ways to prepare for your interview day:

1) **Accept the interview with gratitude.** The first thing to do in preparation for your interview day is to express your gratitude to the medical school, and graciously accept the interview with excitement. Be prompt with your acceptance. Taking longer than necessary can be viewed as lack of interest.

2) **Choose the right outfit.** Whether we like it or not, appearance matters. What to wear for an interview has become a divided topic. Some say you should dress con-

servatively (e.g., black, grey, or dark blue outfit), while others say to "be yourself" and wear something that reflects who you are. My personal advice is to dress the part—you want to look as if you could be someone's doctor. Your interviewers should be able to envision you as an excellent physician. If you don't have an appropriate outfit in your wardrobe, buy something. If you can't afford it, then borrow something.

3) **Make your travel plans early.** The medical school application process is rather expensive. You can easily spend up to $4,000, depending on how many programs you apply to. As soon as you confirm your interview, make the necessary arrangements for your transportation and accommodations. Don't pay higher rates unnecessarily because you waited too long to make these purchases. Cut costs where you can.

4) **Do a mock interview.** This one goes without saying. You must practice for the interview. Body language, enunciation, eye contact—these things must be mastered. I recommend you do at least three mock interviews. When the real day comes, you want to feel as comfortable as possible. Your premed advisor should be able to assist with finding mock interview opportunities.

5) **Research the school.** Hopefully, since you applied to the school, you already know a lot about it. Now you need to go deeper. Know the school's values and missions. Learn details pertaining to their student body characteristics (e.g., first-year class size). When they ask you why you want to attend their school, you should have enough of an understanding about the school to answer truthfully.

My challenge to you this week is to do a mock interview

with your accountability buddy. This should be a fun one!

I'd love to hear how your challenge went. Tweet me @DoctorDaleMD #PreMedMondays. I continue to pray for your success, and I look forward to our time together next Monday.

*Dr. Dale*

### THIS WEEK'S ASSIGNMENT

• Meet up with your accountability buddy to do a mock interview.
• Which interview questions were the hardest to answer? Which were the easiest?

# Week 44

# FIVE INTERVIEW QUESTIONS TO PREPARE FOR

*To my premedical friend:*

I won't lie to you—some interviewers are tough. They can make you sweat! The most challenging question I was asked was, "If you could resurrect any two people, who would they be?" Wow! While every interviewer is different, there are some basic questions you must be prepared to answer. Here are five of them:

1) **Why do you want to be a medical doctor?** This age-old question will never be removed from the medical school interview process. You should have a short, and convincing, answer for this question. Expect to be asked this at every interview.

2) **Why are you interested in our medical school?** Medical schools have options. There are more applicants than available positions. When interviewing students, they

want to be sure that you truly want to be there. To provide a good answer for this question, you should have done your research on that medical school. Make sure you can communicate how their institutional mission aligns with your personal mission.

3) **How do you deal with stress?** This question is very important because medical school is stressful. Admission committee members want to be certain that when times get tough, you can overcome them. If you are asked this question, it would be good to provide an example of a stressful situation and the mechanisms you used to overcome it.

4) **Tell me about yourself.** Though this is a simple question, it carries a lot of weight. Prepare your "elevator pitch" (a short, tactful speech that tells your interviewer who you are and why you would be a perfect candidate for their school). Brag, but don't boast. Be humble, but not boring. Remember, this is your moment to shine.

5) **Tell me about this accomplishment you submitted on your application.** Don't mess this one up! Make sure you know your application forward and backward. If you can't describe an accomplishment in detail, then consider excluding it from your application.

My challenge to you this week is to come up with an elevator pitch that answers the question, "Tell me about yourself." Practice this elevator pitch with your accountability buddy.

I'd love to see a one-minute video with your pitch. Post it on your PreMed STAR profile and tweetme @DoctorDaleMD #PreMedMondays. I continue to pray for your success, and I look forward to our time together next Monday.

*Dr. Dale*

## THIS WEEK'S ASSIGNMENT

- How does your elevator pitch answer the question, "Tell me about yourself"?
- Practice this elevator pitch with your accountability buddy.
- Post your elevator pitch video on your PreMed STAR profile.

# Week 45

# FIVE QUESTIONS TO ASK YOUR INTERVIEWER

*To my premedical friend:*

Most of your medical school interviews are going to end with this question: "Now, what questions do you have for me?" Even if you don't have any burning questions, it is important to ask something meaningful. Doing so demonstrates your interest in the school. Here are five questions to consider asking:

1) **What do you like best about this medical school?** This is an indirectly flattering question. Everybody loves to answer a question like this. It gives interviewers a real chance to brag on their medical school and why you should want to attend there. You can't go wrong with this one!

2) **Do most medical students match in one of their top three residency choices?** After medical school, new doctors go on to residency. For most people, the resi-

dency they attend is based on a matching process. In this process, students get to rank residency programs, and residency programs get to rank students. Through a detailed algorithm, a match is made. You want to know if most students are matching in one of their top three choices. If so, this is a good sign. Asking this question will demonstrate to your interviewer that you are dedicated and understand the entire medical training process.

3) **What research opportunities are available for medical students?** Most first-year medical students are uncertain if they will conduct research during medical school or as a physician. Even if you are not interested in research now, this might change. Medical schools certainly want researchers. They are interested in generating new understandings of how the world works, and they are looking for students who can help them do this. This is an excellent question for all interviewees to ask.

4) **What do students like to do for fun here?** This is a great question to ask because it demonstrates you are already envisioning yourself as a student at that medical school. Don't be surprised to get an answer such as, "It would be best if you asked that of one of the students." If that is their response, don't think the interviewer is trying to dodge the question. They just want you to hear it directly from the student. Be sure to let them know you'll also touch base with some of the students to find out.

5) **Is it okay if I contact you with any questions?** This question is great for two reasons. First, it gives you a direct connection to faculty members who have given

you permission to contact them. Second, when you contact interviewers, you confirm your interest in their medical school.

My challenge to you this week is to spend a few minutes researching the "residency match." It is important for you to understand how the entire medical training process works. Discuss this with your accountability buddy.

I'd love to hear how your challenge went. Tweet me @DoctorDaleMD #PreMedMondays. I continue to pray for your success, and I look forward to our time together next Monday.

*Dr. Dale*

## THIS WEEK'S ASSIGNMENT
- What did you learn about the medical training process after researching the residency match?
- Discuss your findings with your accountability buddy.

# Week 46

# FIVE THINGS TO DO AFTER INTERVIEW DAY

*To my premedical friend:*

Performing well during the medical school interview is only half the battle. After interview day, you've got to face the latter half. It's time to wrap things up and solidify the great impression you left on them! Here are the five things you should do after every interview day:

1) **Send thank-you notes.** Nowadays, this is most often done via email; however, nothing beats a good old-fashioned handwritten note. You do not have to send this to everybody, but consider sending it to the faculty members who interviewed you. When sending emails, also remember to thank the staff members who coordinated your interview day. Also, send a short thank-you note to any medical students that you connected with.

2) **Take notes about what you liked and what you didn't**

**like.** Depending on how many interviews you attend, it's possible that you'll confuse characteristics and events at the various schools. Take notes at the end of every interview day so you'll be able to review them when making your final decision. Documenting events from each interview will also make it possible for you to send meaningful thank-you messages.

3) **Evaluate your performance.** Consider each interview as an opportunity for improvement. Think back to how you answered certain questions, shook hands, and interacted with various medical staff. What did you do well? What do you need to improve prior to your next interview?

4) **Reevaluate your budget.** The interview trail is expensive, and it's easy to go above your budget. The last thing you want to happen is to come up short and not be able to afford your last few interviews. Some students end up canceling interviews as the season progresses. Make sure you have sufficient funds to continue through the application process.

5) **Prepare for the next one.** It's extremely important that you don't lose momentum on the interview trail. It can be exhausting, and you must be an active participant throughout the entire process. No matter how much you liked the school you just interviewed with, keep in mind that there are no guarantees and you shouldn't put all your eggs in one basket.

My challenge to you this week is to draft a brief thank-you email that you can send following the interview day. Polish it up nicely, and save it in a file for later use.

I'd love to hear how your challenge went. Tweet me

@DoctorDaleMD #PreMedMondays. I continue to pray for your success, and I look forward to our time together next Monday.

*Dr. Dale*

## THIS WEEK'S ASSIGNMENT

- Draft a brief thank-you email that you can send following the interview day.
- After you polish it up and save it, share the email with your accountability buddy.

# Week 47

# PERSONAL ACCOUNTABILITY

*To my premedical friend:*

This letter may seem a bit harsh, but don't be offended. Sometimes mentors are afraid to say the things that need to be said. We worry too much about hurting your feelings and in the process neglect to do what is in your best interest. This week, I need to give it to you straight. If you don't become a doctor, in most cases, it's nobody's fault but your own. I should also mention that for many of you, the premedical journey will teach you that medicine isn't your cup of tea. This is a blessing in disguise as it can help you find your true calling.

I've been mentoring premedical students long enough to have heard just about every excuse. *But Dr. Dale, you don't understand how much my teacher hates me. I had to take care of my sick parents. I got ill and was hospitalized.* When my mentees share these things with me in confidence, I truly do hurt right alongside them. In many instances, these are real and valid issues. The unfortunate thing, however, is that life doesn't stop because you are pursuing a career in medicine.

The clock continues to tick, and bad things continue to happen. Why did you get sick, but your friends didn't? Only God can answer this. Had you stayed healthy, you would have gotten better grades.

Here's something you need you to understand: Even though life's curveballs come at you fast, you are still the one with the bat in your hands. Nobody else can swing for you. Think about this from the perspective of your future patients. They won't care that you lost a loved one during your premedical years. That may sound bad, but it's true. All they care about it is whether or not you are capable of delivering the care they need. When it comes to your ability to take care of patients, there are no excuses. Either you are good at it or you are not. And if you are not, your patients won't care why—they'll just find another doctor.

I want you to be mentally tough. There are no excuses. We all face challenges, and those who overcome them will be rewarded with the white coat. Something else you need to know is that medical schools are more concerned with *how* you have overcome hardships and grown from them than the actual hardships themselves. Let's say that you have been diagnosed with a medical condition during college. That's unfortunate, and can truly hinder your performance. But if you are able to demonstrate how you successfully took on that challenge, it'll give you the upper hand when applying to medical school.

Life will continue to throw you curveballs, and when they come, swing hard! If you miss, that's okay because you've got another chance at bat. If you nail that one, it's going out of the park.

My challenge to you this week is to identify one excuse that has been holding you back from peak performance. Everybody has one. Are you committed to having no more excuses?

I'd love to hear how your challenge went. Tweet me @DoctorDaleMD #PreMedMondays. I continue to pray for your success, and I look forward to our time together next Monday.

*Dr. Dale*

## THIS WEEK'S ASSIGNMENT

- What is one excuse that has been holding you back from peak performance?
- How can you overcome this excuse?

# Week 48

# FIVE COURSES TO CONSIDER TAKING BEFORE YOU GRADUATE

*To my premedical friend:*

There are two ways to go about choosing your classes. The first is to take the minimum number of prerequisites required to apply and enroll in medical school. The second is to take extra courses that will further prepare you for medical school. I suggest you do the latter. Yes, it is true that your prerequisites will provide a basic foundation of knowledge, but you don't want to be struggling in your first year of med school. Colleges offer these courses for a reason, and I encourage you to take advantage of them. These are five courses to consider taking before starting medical school:

1) **Medical Terminology.** This course will provide you with an excellent foundation for clinical medicine. You will learn the root word meanings of many terms used by doctors and other healthcare providers. Trust me, it is

easy to get stuck in a dictionary early in medical school. Taking medical terminology will significantly reduce the time you spend looking up words.

2) **Medical Microbiology.** Microbiology is a rather difficult course in medical school. There are tons of viruses, bacteria, and fungi that you are expected to know in detail. Give yourself a head start by taking this course prior to medical school.

3) **Pharmacology.** Interestingly, this course is often overlooked by premeds. Doctors prescribe medications all the time, and many of your nights in medical school will be spent learning them. Life as a medical student will certainly be easier if you have a basic knowledge of pharmacology.

4) **Histology.** This is another course that you will be required to take in medical school. Histology is a challenging topic, and you will spend quite some time on it. If your undergraduate campus has a good histology professor, I strongly encourage you to consider taking this course. Also, histology courses tend to overlap with pathology, so you'll get a two for one!

5) **Anatomy.** Yes, of course anatomy. This is the quintessential medical school course and is often among the first things you are expected to master. If you begin medical school with a solid foundation in anatomy, you are likely to perform well early on. This will boost your confidence for future courses.

My challenge to you this week is to review your premedical courses and see whether there is space to add at least one of these courses.

I'd love to hear how your challenge went. Tweet me

@DoctorDaleMD #PreMedMondays. I continue to pray for your success, and I look forward to our time together next Monday.

*Dr. Dale*

**THIS WEEK'S ASSIGNMENT**
- Review your premedical courses.
- Where can you find space to add at least one of these courses?

# Week 49

# FIVE WAYS TO PAY FOR MEDICAL SCHOOL

*To my premedical friend:*

People love talking about how much money we make as physicians. However, the debt we incur isn't nearly as popular of a topic. Medical school is expensive. Correction, medical school is very expensive. It's in your best interest to plan ahead, so you can minimize the amount of debt you will have upon graduation. Here are five ways to pay for medical school:

1) **Loans**. This is the most common way students pay for medical school. Many young doctors begin their careers with $100,000 to $400,000 worth of debt. Yes, this is an alarming number, but remember that your education is an investment. By the same token, you should also remember not to take out more money than you need. Interest is a real thing, and one day, the reapers are coming back for their money.

2) **Scholarships**. Every medical student desires to have

their school tuition paid by someone else. There are numerous scholarships out there for which you can apply. The key is you must be aggressive and diligent in finding them. Every dollar helps!

3) **Employment.** I typically do not advise medical students to work during medical school. There are exceptions, however. Jobs that demand little time and effort are typically okay. Tutoring jobs also tend to be okay because you are studying in the process. Other than jobs such as those, I would caution you not to work during this period of life. Med school is hard enough as is. You don't want distractions to make it harder.

4) **Government grants.** Depending on your financial situation, you might qualify for some government grants to help fund medical school. Like scholarships, you do not want to pass on this free money. Do your research to see if you qualify for any of these opportunities. If so, take advantage!

5) **Parents.** Some people are fortunate to have parents who can help pay for medical school. If you are one of those individuals, great! Be sure to give your parents a great big hug for helping you out in such a huge way. Don't take it for granted. That's a big deal!

My challenge to you this week is to look up the tuition for five medical schools you are interested in. Were the costs what you expected them to be?

I'd love to hear how your challenge went. Tweet me @DoctorDaleMD #PreMedMondays. I continue to pray for your success, and I look forward to our time together next Monday.

*Dr. Dale*

**THIS WEEK'S ASSIGNMENT**
- What is the tuition for five medical schools you are interested in?
- Were the costs higher or lower than what you expected?

# Week 50

# FIVE REASONS TO CONSIDER A GAP YEAR

*To my premedical friend:*

For a variety of reasons, premedical students sometimes take a year or more "off" before starting medical school. It's not really time off since they are doing other things that can strengthen their application. This period is referred to as a "gap" year(s). Gap years allow you to explore other opportunities and further develop yourself. Here are five reasons to consider taking a gap year:

1) **To earn an extra degree.** Many students get a master's degree during their gap years. This is great because it provides you with an additional knowledge base, which may be beneficial throughout your medical career. And of course, medical schools look favorably upon students who have some graduate-level education prior to applying.

2) **To earn money.** For the past few years of your life, you've probably been living on a tight student budget. It's difficult to imagine how you will survive financially during medical school. Gap years allow you to work and potentially have a decent income before applying to medical school. Beyond the money, the work experience itself is a wonderful perk.

3) **To reapply to medical school.** Let's say you didn't get accepted the first time around. But applying without success doesn't mean you are finished. This is the perfect opportunity to refocus and try again. If it's your dream, give it a fair shot! Use your gap year(s) to improve your candidacy.

4) **To take a well-deserved break.** Hopefully, for the past four years or so, you've worked hard to earn good grades. It is reasonable to want a break from the classroom environment. When you start medical school, you'll hit the ground running. You don't want to start this journey burned out.

5) **To confirm that a career in medicine is right for you.** Pursuing a career in medicine is a major commitment. This path will demand your time, money, and your heart. Before you commit to it, you need to be certain it's what you want. If you don't have adequate clinical experience, and feel the need for more confirmation, consider taking a gap year to make certain medicine is right for you.

My challenge to you this week is to find someone who has taken, or is thinking about taking, a gap year and ask them why. If you don't know anyone personally, you'll find some on PreMed STAR.

I'd love to hear how your challenge went. Tweet me

@DoctorDaleMD #PreMedMondays. I continue to pray for your success, and I look forward to our time together next Monday.

*Dr. Dale*

## THIS WEEK'S ASSIGNMENT

- Find someone who has taken, or is thinking about taking, a gap year.
- What were some of the positives and negatives of that person's experience?

# Week 51

# FIVE REASONS WHY IT'S WORTH THE WAIT

*To my premedical friend:*

Staying motivated along this journey can be difficult, but I want to assure you that it is all worth it. Don't be fooled by those who would have you believe doctors aren't happy. I'll tell you from firsthand experience that I'm very happy. I'll also tell you that my physician friends appear happy as well. Always remember that there is light at the end of the tunnel. Here are five reasons your hard work and patience are worth the wait:

1) **You become someone special.** Hard work is never about the things you get as a result. Material things come and go, but what lasts is the person you become. Your initiation into medical training is similar to boot camp. It takes a great deal of discipline for you to make it through successfully. This process molds you into someone special. Someone you couldn't have become otherwise.

2) **You are entering a secure field.** The great thing about being a doctor is that your skills are useful anywhere you go. At some point, we all need healthcare. That being the case, the demand for clinicians won't be slowing down anytime soon. Your premedical and medical school training will add so much value to you as a person, which is hard to lose. If you continue to practice medicine under the tenants you learn along the way, you'll have job security for life (assuming you are physically and mentally fit to care for patients).

3) **The pay's not bad.** Doctors make a lot of money. The time spent training, the debt incurred, and the significance of what we do justify our price tag. While you are in medical school, many of your friends will be working and earning real paychecks. Don't let that bother you, because your checks will come soon enough, and hopefully you'll be satisfied with them.

4) **People are depending on you.** The driving force behind everything I do is the knowledge that other people are depending on me. Your premedical days are worth the effort because your future patients are depending on you to become their doctor. When you emerge on the other side of training in a bright white coat, they're counting on you to be an excellent physician.

5) **It's your dream.** You haven't read these letters to simply pass time. No, you did so because you dream of becoming a medical doctor. You'll have trials and tribulations during these premedical and medical school years, but your dream is worth it all.

My challenge to you this week is to write down five character traits you hope to develop or strengthen during your premedical years. Discuss them with your accountability buddy, and remember, it's the person you become that makes all this worth it!

I'd love to hear how your challenge went. Tweet me @DoctorDaleMD #PreMedMondays. I continue to pray for your success, and I look forward to our time together next Monday.

*Dr. Dale*

## THIS WEEK'S ASSIGNMENT

• List the five character traits you hope to develop or strengthen as a premed.

1)

2)

3)

4)

5)

• Discuss your list with your accountability buddy.

# Week 52

# MY BEST WISHES FOR YOU

*To my premedical friend:*

Can you believe it has been one year already? Time certainly does fly. I've enjoyed writing these letters to you, and I would like to leave you with some final thoughts for your future.

I hope you've become a stronger person over this past year. I've written to you to encourage you on your premedical journey, but my greater passion is contributing to your development as a human being. Most of the principles and values I have written to you were not taught to me by medical doctors. They are not at all specific to medicine. Remember that first and foremost, you are a human being; your identity is not solely defined by being a doctor.

A mentor of mine once told me something that has stuck with me all of these years. He said, "Dale, you are more than a doctor." Those simple words changed my life. I want you to be aware of this same truth. You are more than a premedical student, and you will be more than a doctor. Be excellent at life!

I hope you will take the time to mentor and encourage others. The wise master teacher once said that the greatest in the kingdom is the servant of all (see Matthew 20:26–27; 23:11). Your success in life isn't determined by what you have, it's determined by what you give.

There are many people in this world waiting for someone like you to come along and give them the encouragement they need. They're waiting for you to be their hope when there is none. You never know who you'll influence. What you say to a younger student today might be the very thing that leads that person to become the greatest doctor, president, or artist the world has ever known.

Let this book be an example to you. Take the principles and values I have shared with you and master them. Mentor someone and share your knowledge. Serve others! There's more fulfillment in doing that than you could ever imagine.

I hope you know how much I love you all. This book of letters truly comes from my heart. Every day, I give my all to help develop people, and move them one step closer to their dreams. It's not easy. I'm met with many "no's" and rejections. But I don't stop, because I am doing it for you.

I know that many of you don't have mentors in your life, and I have done my best in these letters to be a mentor to you. This means a lot to me, and I do not take the responsibility lightly. The fact that you would take the time to listen to my guidance and trust in me is overwhelming. My eyes are literally tearing up as I am writing this letter. I am imagining how much you've grown this past year. I feel like I've been there walking alongside you the entire way.

This week, I leave you with no challenge. Just my well wishes and most sincere prayers for your success. I'd love to hear how you've grown during our time together. Please tweet me @DoctorDaleMD #PreMedMondays. Thank you for letting me walk this journey with you. I will continue to do my best to serve you.

Dr. Dale

p.s. I leave you with the words of my favorite teacher. Please, let this be your mindset throughout your career and life.

"The greatest among you shall be your servant."

—JESUS CHRIST, MATTHEW 23:11 ESV

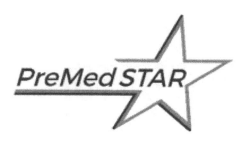

Be sure to join the online community for premedical students. Download the app for free in your app store. With PreMed STAR, you can network with other premeds, manage your resume/curriculum vitae, share class notes, get recruited by medical schools, and much more.

**www.PreMedSTAR.com**

# SEND ME YOUR PHOTO!

*Thank you for reading my book! I pray it has transformed you in some way for the better. If it did, here's how you can let me know. Take a nice photo (it's ok to get creative) and send it to me with a brief statement of how this book has impacted you. I'll be sharing these photos on my website and social media platforms, so we can support each other in developing tomorrow's leaders in medicine.*

Email the photo and your social media
names to me at:

## Dale@DoctorDaleMD.com

*Again, thank you so very much for reading my book!*

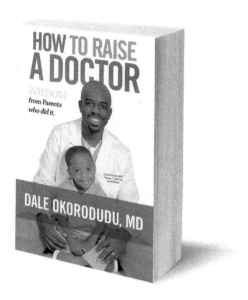

In *How to Raise a Doctor: Wisdom from Parents who Did It!*, Dale Okorodudu, MD draws from the lessons of parents who strategically and successfully guided their children to become medical doctors. It turns out that for many of these parents, it really wasn't that difficult.

After interviewing 75 parents of physicians, Dr. Dale provides their most essential instructions for raising doctors in this practical and powerful book. These are key strategies that you can begin applying today!

From childhood character traits, daily habits, and parenting styles, to the medical school application process, How to Raise a Doctor covers it all. But raising a doctor isn't the ultimate goal. Raising a leader, is! Regardless of what profession your child decides to work in, this book will show you how to raise the leader your child was born to be!

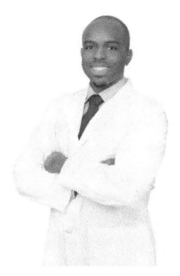

**Faith. Family. Friends.**

# MEET DR. DALE

Dale Okorodudu, MD is a husband, dad, and physician. He is the author of *How to Raise a Doctor* and the founder of PreMed STAR. Dr. Dale's passion lies in developing the physician leaders of tomorrow.

To learn more about Dr. Dale,
visit **www.DoctorDaleMD.com**.

www.facebook.com/DoctorDaleMD

www.twitter.com/DoctorDaleMD

www.DoctorDaleMD.com